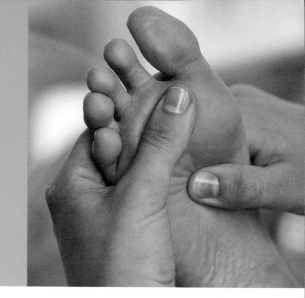

5-minute
massages

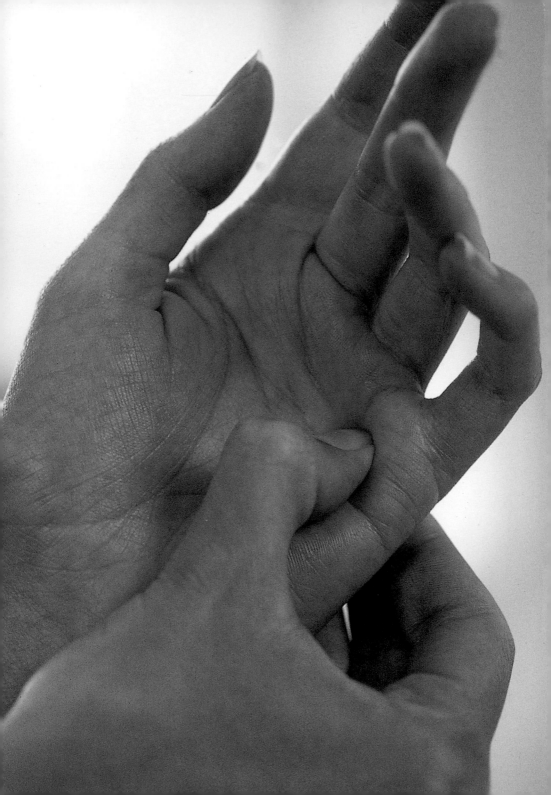

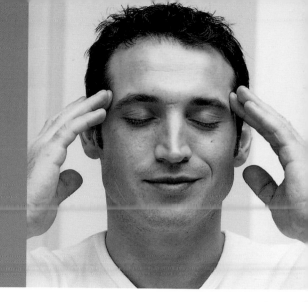

5-minute
massages

fingertip
techniques for
over 30 common
complaints

hamlyn

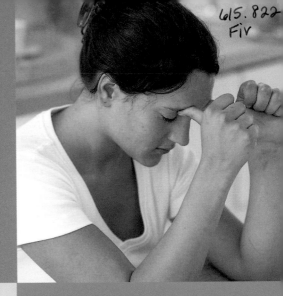

A Pyramid Paperback

First published in Great Britain in 2006 by
Hamlyn, a division of Octopus Publishing Group Ltd
2–4 Heron Quays, London E14 4JP

Copyright © Octopus Publishing Group Limited 2006

Distributed in the United States and Canada by
Sterling Publishing Co., Inc.
387 Park Avenue South, New York, NY 10016-8810

Some of the material in this publication has been
previously published in the following titles: *Healing
Massage, Head Massage, Reflexology and
Acupressure, Thai Bodywork, Home Health Spa,
Hand Reflexology, Home Health Massage, Natural
Highs for Body and Soul.*

ISBN-13: 978-0-600-61441-8
ISBN-10: 0-600-61441-7

A CIP catalogue record for this book is available from
the British Library

Printed and bound in China

10 9 8 7 6 5 4 3 2 1

Notes

While the advice and information in this book is
believed to be accurate, neither the author nor the
publisher will be responsible for any injury, losses,
damages, actions, proceedings, claims, demands,
expenses and costs (including legal costs or
expenses) incurred or in any way arising out of
following the exercises in this book.

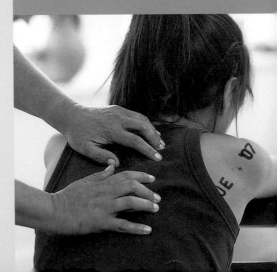

Contents

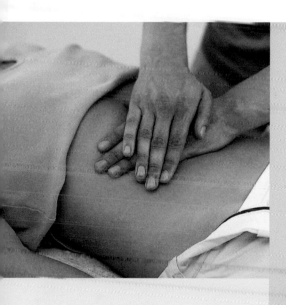

What is massage?

Massage therapy has evolved out of one of our most basic desires – to touch and be touched. By manipulating the body's soft tissues with specific techniques to promote or restore health, it is possible to use your hands to detect and treat problems in the muscles, ligaments and tendons. And research shows that massage can help with everything from stress relief and related conditions such as insomnia and depression to convalescence after surgery.

To the Ancient Greek and Roman physicians, massage was one of the principal means of healing and relieving pain. In c.400 BCE, Hippocrates – the father of modern medicine – wrote: 'The physician must be experienced in many things, but assuredly in rubbing... For rubbing can bind a joint that is too loose, and loosen a joint that is too rigid.' Practised for thousands of years, now in the 21st century massage has become a mainstream and popular complementary therapy. It is used throughout the world by people of all ages and walks of life, and has a very important role to play in maintaining a healthy lifestyle.

In today's fast-paced, 24/7 society, massage can play an invaluable role in boosting wellbeing with the introduction of simple techniques into everyday life. Although massage is still often seen as a luxury for those with time on their hands, it doesn't have to mean lying in a darkened room listening to whale music for an hour, while paying someone a large sum of money. In fact, there are quick and easy ways to make the most of massage that take no longer than five minutes, which you can do to a partner or perform on yourself while sitting at your desk or watching television.

How does it work?

There are many different types of massage, using a variety of approaches and techniques. All basic massage techniques, even if done as a quick routine for five minutes, have been shown to stimulate physical and emotional healing in two ways:

- **The mechanical effects of massage,** which including pressing, squeezing and moving the soft tissues of the body, relaxing the muscles and stimulating the circulation so that blood flows freely, carrying oxygen and nutrients to wherever they are needed.

- **The reflex action,** which is triggered in one part of the body as an involuntary reaction to the stimulation of another part – for example, a relaxing back massage can also have the effect of easing leg pain.

Massaging the skin also stimulates the immune system and improves overall health. Some experts even believe that we could replace 90 per cent of mainstream medicine with a simple weekly massage.

Those massage disciplines that have an Eastern background, such as reflexology, acupressure, Thai massage and shiatsu, also believe that the physical pressure of massage has an effect on an inner energy, often known as *chi* or *ki*, that circulates within our bodies. This energy runs through channels, sometimes called meridians, or *sen* lines, and pressing on certain points on the hands, feet, or elsewhere on the body can cause the healing of organs or body areas at a deep level.

The benefits of massage

Stress in the 21st century is one of the main causes of poor health. Slowing down, switching off and stepping off the treadmill of life isn't easy. All too often as the pace hots up, we respond with the reflex action of tensing our bodies just to 'hold on' in order to protect our dipping energy resources. Our bodies become heavier, weighed down with all these responsibilities. The inevitable effects of stressful living will eventually have a serious impact on our health.

This is where massage comes in. Relaxation and massage are both methods of allowing our systems time to calm down and recuperate.

Massage provides a great boost for general health and wellbeing, improving the workings of both mind and body, but it also helps relieve certain commonly occurring conditions. Often all you need is a simple, five-minute routine to see a noticeable improvement in the following ways.

- **Nervous system** Massage helps soothe, relax and invigorate the nervous system, zapping fatigue and deep-rooted stresses and strains.

- **Circulation** Massage greatly improves circulation, thus helping to eradicate the problem of cold feet and hands as well as stiffness in the joints.

- **Mental faculties** By unblocking the channels that carry the flow of energy through the body, head massage increases the supply of oxygen to the brain and is a great way of releasing tension. Soothing the senses through massage helps banish unwanted thoughts and curbs the tendency to daydream, leaving the mind clearer, calmer and more focused.

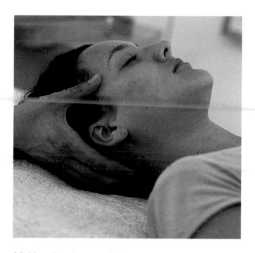

Making time in your daily life for massage can help ease stress and tension, and also treat a variety of specific ailments.

- **Everyday ailments and conditions** Touching pressure points can relieve everyday problems such as asthma, bronchitis, constipation, indigestion and skin disorders.

- **Depression and anxiety** A quick massage routine can help calm and soothe the mind, and prevent panic attacks. It will help lift your mood day by day.

- **Headaches and migraines** Massage can readjust the balance of pressures in the head, clearing sinuses, de-stressing neck and shoulder muscles and relieving eyestrain.

- **Women's health problems** Massage can also help to relieve the symptoms of PMT and the menopause, as well as ease menstrual pain.

Getting started

Massage is easy to learn. Follow your instincts and you will be able to sense where to touch, how to touch and for how long. It is not, however, a good idea to try to massage if you are feeling stressed or tense, or if you are not in good health, as your energy levels will be low.

In the following pages we will be introducing some of the most popular forms of massage, and explaining a little about them and how they work. We have then taken over 30 of the most common ailments and shown how they can be treated with different quick and easy types of massage. Some of the techniques involve self-massage; others require two people, known as a giver and receiver. Some massages can be done anywhere, such as sitting at a desk or on a train or plane, while others require you to lie down in comfort. Either way, each routine should take no longer than five minutes and will leave you feeling significantly better. We have also included 'quick fixes' for those especially stressful times when you need emergency relief or an instant lift.

Oils for massage

Most massage treatments require the use of a lubricant to allow your hands to work smoothly and evenly over the skin without breaking the rhythm. This usually takes the form of oil, although lotions and creams can also be used. Use just a thin film, which will be absorbed into the skin after the treatment. You can use sunflower, grapeseed or vegetable oils.

You may be tempted to buy aromatherapy oils, but many are concentrated and have contraindications, so unless you are a trained aromatherapist, stick to oils such as lavender or chamomile, which can be used sparingly in neat form. Other essential oils should not be applied neat to the skin: always mix with a carrier oil, such as vegetable oil, in the ratio of 1 drop essential oil to 2 ml (scant ½ teaspoon) carrier oil.

Preparing for massage

For a self-massage, simply make sure that you are dressed appropriately and that your finger nails are not too long. Remove any jewellery and apply hand cream to soothe rough skin if necessary. If you are giving a massage, wear comfortable clothes and footwear, and make sure you and the receiver are feeling relaxed.

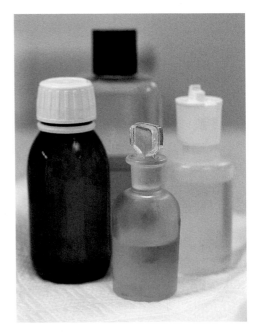

Choose from scented aromatherapy oils, basic carrier oils and pre-blended massage oils, now widely available.

Creating a relaxed environment

Ideally, the room should be comfortably warm so that you (or both you and the receiver, if you are giving a massage) can relax. Try to avoid distractions such as a blaring television or radio on in the background, or children running around. However, you could have some music playing, as relaxing background music can have a soothing effect. It is also a good idea to disconnect the phone and turn off your mobile – and prepare to relax.

Depending on the time of day, subdued lights such as table lamps will set the right tone. Natural light can be good for the daytime, especially the morning, when you might choose an invigorating massage, and in the evening you may wish to create a special mood with candlelight. Choose a time when you can really relax and re-energize.

If you are giving a massage, prepare the massage area, whether it be blankets or a mat on the floor, or a treatment table. Have towels and pillows ready for extra comfort.

When not to massage

In general, massage is safe. Nevertheless, there are certain guidelines that should be observed, and it is best to avoid massaging anyone in the following circumstances:

- If they are weak or clinically exhausted.

- If they have a high temperature or are suffering from a contagious disease.

- If they are suffering from an infectious skin complaint, such as scabies, herpes or warts.

- If they have a serious medical condition, such as cancer, a heart disorder or thrombosis.

- If they have had surgery; also not for 12 months following major procedures – scar tissue should then be fully healed.

- If they are in the first trimester of pregnancy; thereafter, avoid very deep pressure, particularly on the lower back and inside leg from ankle to groin.

- If there are skin problems, such as scar tissue, bruising, tender or inflamed areas and varicose veins; instead of working directly on them, work with care above the site and on other unaffected areas.

- If they have had a recent fracture, sprain or strain (in these cases, work one joint above the site).

It is also not advisable to massage anyone who has recently eaten a heavy meal or has been drinking quantities of alcohol, as this will make the experience very uncomfortable and may produce unpleasant after-effects. The general rule is to trust your own common sense.

Types of massage

The following section introduces the six main forms of therapeutic
massage featured in this book, both Western and Eastern in
origins and traditions. The underlying approach to healing that
each of these therapies takes is explained in simple terms and
the basic techniques they use clearly demonstrated. Once you
have taken a few moments to familiarize yourself with the
principles involved, you will be ready to put them to practical use
in improving your everyday wellbeing.

Western massage

Western massage is the most modern form of massage and is based on Swedish massage, which was first developed at the beginning of the 19th century. However, touch in the form of massage has been practised for thousands of years and its effects have been well researched, providing us with undeniable evidence that massage is good for us in easing aches and pains and promoting a calmer, healthier and happier lifestyle.

How it works

Massage sends messages to the brain and back again – some stimulating, others calming. Touch is known to increase the level of oxytocin, the hormone that makes us stop what we are doing and relax, which in our fast-paced modern society is necessary to restore balance in our lives.

A quick massage routine can also be used more specifically to relieve many complaints, such as stress and stress-related conditions, insomnia, depression and circulation problems. It can also help relieve aching strained muscles and the inflammation associated with arthritis, as well as irritable bowel syndrome and constipation, which are both very common ailments in the West.

If you are massaging someone else, then a two-way flow is involved, and for this to work the giver of the massage must be prepared to give and the receiver must allow them to do so.

Techniques

These are the most frequently used techniques in the treatment of the ailments featured in this book, and are the easiest to deliver.

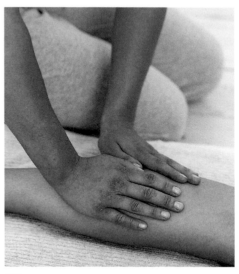
Effleurage

Effleurage

The most simple and useful massage stroke, this involves touching or stroking the body lightly and rhythmically. Use it anywhere on the body, though it is particularly good on the back and chest.

Firm, brisk massage strokes improve the circulation, while gentle rhythmic strokes stimulate the lymph glands and help eliminate body wastes. Slower strokes can ease tense muscles, reduce stress, lower blood pressure and generally relax someone.

Petrissage

This involves pressing, squeezing and rolling the muscles, as well as more specific techniques of kneading and wringing. It is useful for deeper massage, but should be used only after the muscles have been warmed up with effleurage.

It is particularly good on the shoulders and fleshy areas of the body such as the thighs. Petrissage releases tension from stiff muscles, improves blood and oxygen circulation and helps eliminate metabolic wastes. It also breaks down fatty deposits, so that they can be eliminated more easily.

Kneading

Place both hands on the body with your fingers pointing away from you. Press into the body with the palm of one hand, the thumb outstretched, and pick up the flesh between your thumb and fingers. Squeeze and roll it towards the resting hand in a side-to-side action, like kneading dough. Release and do the same with the other hand, rhythmically squeezing and releasing. Apply light or deep pressure. Work your way up the muscle, keeping contact with both hands in a continuous rhythmic movement.

Wringing

This is similar to kneading, but you keep the thumb closed to the fingers and work alternately backwards and forwards in a continuous flow, lifting the skin with one hand and pushing it away with the other, as if you were wringing out a wet towel.

Knuckling

Make loose fists with your hands and uncurl your fingers so that the middle section of each finger rests on the skin. Move your fingers in a circular motion to give a rippling effect.

Use it on the soles of the feet, palms of the hands, shoulders and chest. Its effects are to increase the blood flow to the specific body area and release muscle tension, particularly when worked deeply.

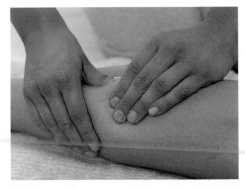

Petrissage – kneading

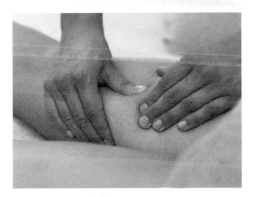

Petrissage – wringing

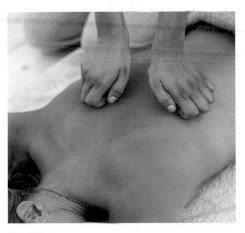

Knuckling

Reflexology

Reflexology is a type of massage therapy that involves applying pressure to points on the feet and hands. By working on a particular point, it is possible to stimulate energy by a reflex action to a related muscle or organ and encourage healing. Learning to treat yourself with reflexology is very relaxing.

Reflexologists believe that all parts of the body are connected by subtle energy, which flows down the body from the head to the feet through ten zones (also known as channels or vessels). When there is illness or discomfort, the channels become blocked and the flow of energy is disturbed. Working on the hands and/or feet unblocks the channels, allows energy to flow and restores the balance, all of which relaxes the body, enhances the circulation and relieves uncomfortable symptoms.

Relief can be almost immediate in many cases. Reflexologists believe that the body heals itself from the inside to the outside. If symptoms have been suppressed by medical treatment, they may return briefly, which is why they sometimes become worse for a while after the first few treatments, before the reflexology starts to work.

How it works

Reflexology is a holistic complementary therapy. Its purpose is to treat the whole person rather than the symptom. Working exclusively on one part of the body may get the energy moving in that area only to have it stagnate elsewhere, so a reflexology session normally starts by working on the whole foot, or hand, in order to treat the entire person, before concentrating on the area that needs extra help. Wherever possible, it is best to give both feet or hands a full treatment.

Techniques

Start and finish each section with long, smooth strokes down the foot, working towards the ankle. Do the same after working on any sensitive areas, to ease discomfort and draw excess energy out of the area. Most reflex points are worked with the fingertips and the edge of the thumb, using firm pressure.

You will probably use all the following methods during the course of a treatment. When working on your own foot, thumb- and finger-walking and rotation on a point are the easiest methods to use.

Thumb- and finger-walking or caterpillar

Flex your thumb or finger at the first joint, while simultaneously sliding it forwards – similar to the movement of a caterpillar.

Hooking

Form a 'hook' by bending your thumb, the thumb tip being the end of the hook. Using your four fingers as a lever, use this hook to gouge into a specific reflex point on your foot or hand, then work the area until any deposits are destroyed or pain subsides. The idea is to hook in and push up and down medially or laterally, imagining that the specific reflex point is hidden and must be located and stimulated. Hold a steady pressure for five seconds, then gradually release the thumb.

Rotation on a point

Keep your thumb or index finger on one spot and rotate it with slightly increased pressure in order to activate that point.

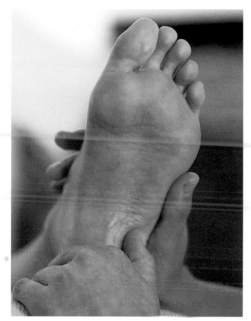

Thumb-walking or caterpillar

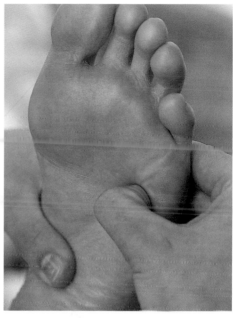

Hooking

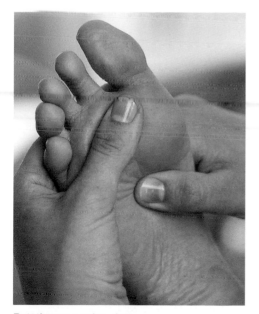

Rotation on a point – foot

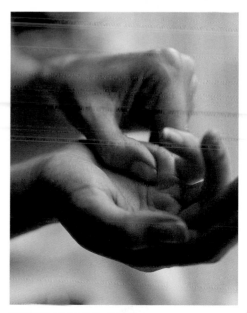

Rotation on a point – hand

▶

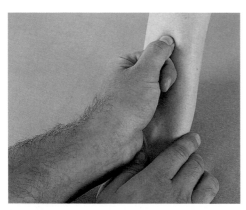

Butterfly

Butterfly

Bend the index finger so that both finger joints are closed. Place the thumb on the finger joint so that the tip overrides the joint of the index finger as a supporting bridge. Depress and raise the thumb tip over a reflex area.

Bird's beak

Press the tip of your thumb against your fingertip to form a 'beak'; this action involves forming the beginning of a pinch, but not actually pinching. Keeping the tip of your thumb pressed against your finger, begin walking the tip of the index finger over the reflex area, leaving the thumb behind. Continue over the area, moving caterpillar style.

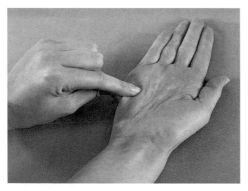

Bird's beak

Tearing

Used in hand reflexology, this movement is like the caterpillar, but in order to reach the more hidden or tough, resistant reflexes, you have to really tear, usually laterally, to hit the reflex point; the firmer you tear, the greater the stimulation. The move is more about what you are trying to tear – a very thick material – since it never gets truly torn.

The zones

The body is divided into ten zones, numbered from one to five on each side of the body. The zones run from the tips of the toes to the head and back down to the fingertips, each one starting at a toe and at a finger or thumb and linking all parts of the body within one zone. Applying pressure to the hands and feet will stimulate the flow of energy throughout the corresponding zone. The longitudinal zones extend through the body from head to toe and from front to back.

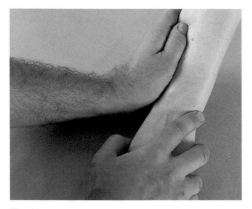

Tearing

The zones

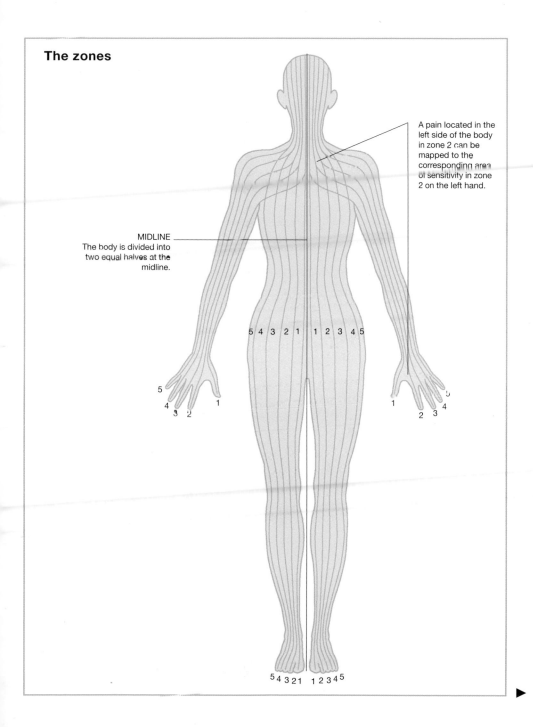

A pain located in the left side of the body in zone 2 can be mapped to the corresponding area of sensitivity in zone 2 on the left hand.

MIDLINE
The body is divided into two equal halves at the midline.

5 4 3 2 1   1 2 3 4 5

5
4
3 2   1

1   5
4
2 3

5 4 3 2 1   1 2 3 4 5

The reflex systems

Reflexologists see the whole body reflected onto the hands or the feet, so most of the body is represented on each hand or foot. Some organs are represented twice, with a small reflex point within a larger area for the organ. A treatment generally includes pressing or hooking firmly on a specific reflex point for about five seconds and also thumb- or finger-walking over the whole organ area. Always work forwards, away from yourself; this frees the flow of energy to remove blockages. Keep changing position or turning the hand or foot in order to avoid working back towards yourself.

When you are working on yourself, you will soon get used to moving your hands and feet around to allow for this manoeuvre.

Head and neck area

The brain and central nervous system are centred on the big toe. Covering all the toes will work these, plus the face and the glands, muscles and sensory organs in that area. Work this part of the foot to treat disorders such as headaches, migraine, insomnia, stress and problems of the eyes, ears and nose.

Chest area

Stretching across the ball of the foot is an area that includes both the respiratory system (disorders such as asthma, bronchitis, hay fever and allergic reactions) and the cardiovascular system (disorders of the heart and circulation, including angina, high blood pressure, varicose veins and cold fingers).

REFLEXES OF THE SOLES OF THE FEET

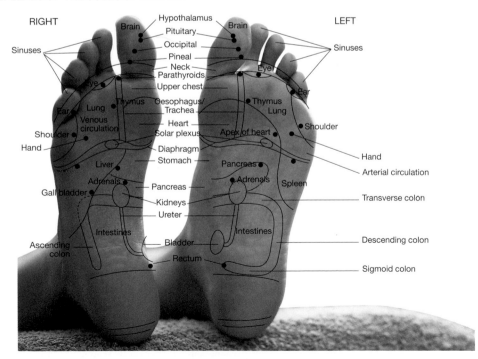

RIGHT — Brain — Hypothalamus — Pituitary — Brain — LEFT

Sinuses — Occipital — Sinuses

Pineal

Neck

Parathyroids

Eye — Upper chest

Thymus — Oesophagus/Trachea — Thymus — Lung — Ear

Lung

Venous circulation — Heart — Shoulder

Shoulder — Solar plexus — Apex of heart

Hand — Diaphragm — Stomach — Pancreas — Hand

Liver — Adrenals — Arterial circulation

Adrenals — Pancreas — Spleen — Transverse colon

Gall bladder — Kidneys

Ureter — Descending colon

Intestines — Intestines

Ascending colon — Bladder — Sigmoid colon

Rectum

Abdomen, digestive and eliminatory systems

These cover the area across each sole below the ball of the foot, as well as most of the instep below that. The area includes the liver, spleen, stomach (found mainly on the left foot), pancreas, gall bladder, colon and rectum. Many of the vital organs are represented in this area, including most of the digestive system, so you can cover most of the organs quite simply by working back and forth across both feet.

Urinary and reproductive systems

These include the bladder, kidneys, adrenal glands, reproductive organs and uterus or prostate. There is a specific point for the latter and the ovary/testis.

URINARY AND REPRODUCTIVE REFLEXES

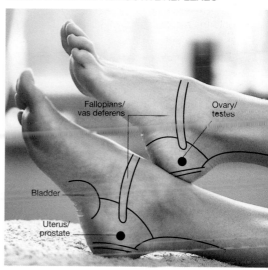

Fallopians/vas deferens

Ovary/testes

Bladder

Uterus/prostate

REFLEXES OF THE TOPS OF THE FEET

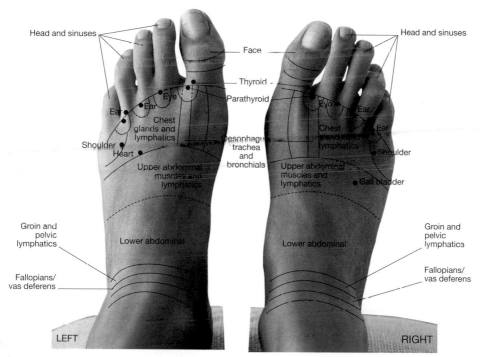

Head and sinuses

Face

Thyroid

Parathyroid

Eye

Ear

Ear

Chest glands and lymphatics

Shoulder

Heart

Oesophagus trachea and bronchials

Upper abdominal muscles and lymphatics

Groin and pelvic lymphatics

Lower abdominal

Fallopians/vas deferens

Head and sinuses

Eye

Ear

Chest glands and lymphatics

Shoulder

Gall bladder

Upper abdominal muscles and lymphatics

Lower abdominal

Groin and pelvic lymphatics

Fallopians/vas deferens

LEFT

RIGHT

Lymphatic system

This system drains wastes from the body's cells with the help of lymph nodes, which are situated throughout the body, with large collections in the chest, groin and armpits. Good lymphatic drainage is essential to help the body cleanse itself from the toxins that have built up within it. It defends the body from foreign bodies such as viruses, bacteria, or fungi.

Endocrine system

Pressure points affecting this system are mainly used when treating hormonal problems. It includes the pituitary (the master gland), the hypothalamus (which connects with the nervous system), thyroid and parathyroids, the thymus, adrenal glands, spleen, pancreas and ovary/testis.

SKELETAL AND SPINAL REFLEXES

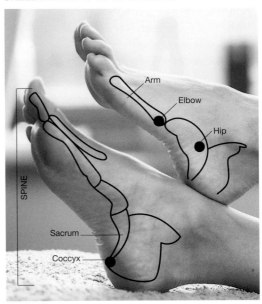

REFLEXES OF THE PALMS OF THE HANDS

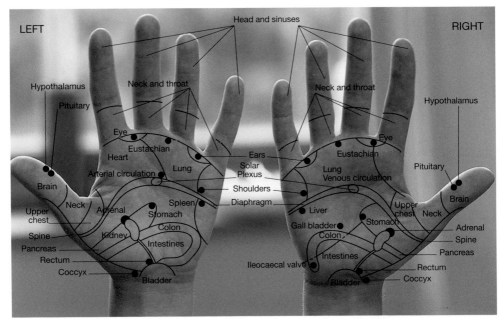

Musculoskeletal system

Work this system to treat problems of the spine, shoulders and neck, repetitive strain injury (RSI), carpal tunnel syndrome, rheumatism and arthritis, among other ailments.

Hand reflexology

This modification of traditional reflexology of the foot comes into its own when conditions don't allow the time or space for working on the feet and also in emergencies. It is also something you can do unobtrusively for yourself when you are out, for example to fend off travel sickness in a car, boat or plane (see page 104).

For people who aren't used to physical therapies, or who feel self-conscious about their feet, a hand treatment offers many of the same benefits as traditional reflexology but in a more acceptable way. Touch itself can be healing,

and hand reflexology offers a very natural and acceptable way of providing a healing touch, using soothing massage-like techniques.

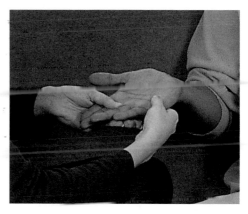

Hand reflexology is a good alternative to treating the feet, especially if the receiver isn't comfortable with having his or her feet touched.

REFLEXES OF THE TOPS OF THE HANDS

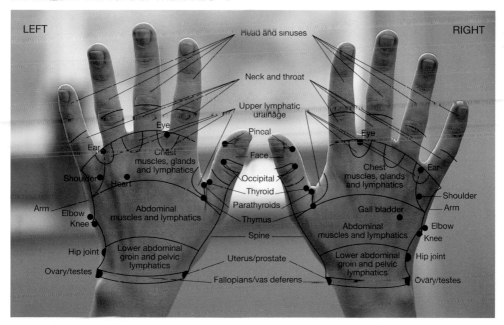

LEFT   RIGHT

Head and sinuses

Neck and throat

Upper lymphatic drainage

Eye — Pineal — Eye

Ear — Chest muscles, glands and lymphatics — Face — Chest muscles, glands and lymphatics — Ear

Shoulder — Heart — Occipital — Shoulder

Thyroid

Arm — Elbow — Abdominal muscles and lymphatics — Parathyroids — Gall bladder — Arm

Knee — Thymus — Abdominal muscles and lymphatics — Elbow

Spine — Knee

Hip joint — Lower abdominal groin and pelvic lymphatics — Uterus/prostate — Lower abdominal groin and pelvic lymphatics — Hip joint

Ovary/testes — Fallopians/vas deferens — Ovary/testes

Acupressure

Acupressure is a practical, hands-on therapy that adapts well to everyday life. It involves pressure point techniques, so is great for those interested in self-help. Finger pressure is used on acupressure points throughout the body to stimulate the flow of *chi* – vital energy that the body runs on. It involves mostly thumb and fingertip pressure, although it can also incorporate massage along the meridians – the body's energy channels.

Acupressure is part of traditional Chinese medicine, having evolved over a period of more than 3,000 years. The belief is that working on one area has a beneficial effect on another area, in the same way as reflexology does. Although it follows a different map – the ancient Chinese meridians rather than zones – most of the principles are the same. There are 22 meridians and 660 pressure points in all. Although acupressure is often described as an offshoot of acupuncture, acupressure probably came first, as people gradually noticed that pressure on certain points on the body relieved pain.

How it works

There are 14 main meridians, six on each side of the body, and one each down the centre of the front and the back. Twelve of these are each connected to one of the internal organs and have a greater effect on that organ.

The meridians are grouped in pairs, one yin and one yang: opposite forces that complement each other, often described as male and female energies. There are two of each of the organ meridians, and they follow identical pathways on the left and right sides of the body.

Stroking or massaging your skin along the route of the meridian is said to help balance the body's systems, and particular points on the meridian are especially beneficial to work on. There are literally hundreds of these acupressure points, but only some of the most valuable and easy to work on ones are included here.

Trigger points are different again. These are tender spots, where acupressure overlaps with anatomy. The value of the trigger point is that it connects with the source of the pain.

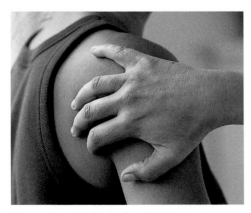

Massaging with the pads of the fingers

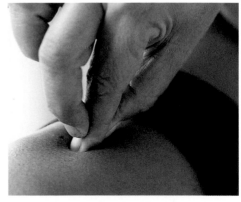

Reinforcing the pressure on a point

Techniques

Press with the flat of your palm when you are working on muscles. Massage with the pads of your fingers, not digging in with the fingertips.

Press into individual points with your index finger, or use your thumb for increased pressure. You can reinforce the pressure by placing the thumb and middle and index fingers together.

Use a light touch over bony areas, which can be painful

On the most sensitive spots, touch with the tips of your middle and index fingers, without applying any pressure.

Using one finger, go in very lightly with a circular movement, without lifting if off the skin. Hold your finger on the point. Reinforce the finger with the thumb and middle finger, so that all three are pressing together.

If there is pain, work above or below it on the same meridian.

The meridians

Lung meridian (Lu) Runs from the top of the chest down to the thumb. Linked with tears and sorrow.

Large intestine meridian (LI) Runs upwards from the index finger to the edge of the nose. Linked with cleansing and detoxifying

Stomach meridian (St) Runs down the body from the head to the second toe. Associated with balancing and nourishing the system.

Spleen meridian (Sp) Runs upwards from the big toe to the armpits. Associated with learning and concentration.

Heart meridian (H) Runs from the top of the arm to the hand. Associated with the mind and long-term memory.

Small intestine meridian (SI) Runs up the arm and shoulder from the little finger to the edge of the jawbone. Linked with the heart.

Bladder meridian (Bl) Runs down the back a couple of finger-widths away from the spine. Linked with transforming fluids.

Kidney meridian (Ki) Goes up the body from the sole of the foot to the top of the chest. The body's energy source, also linked with growth, willpower and short-term memory.

Pericardium meridian (Pc) Runs from the chest to the middle finger. Linked with anxiety and tension.

Triple energizer meridian (TE) Runs from the ring finger to the eyebrow. Linked with regulating warmth and balancing the body's fluid levels between the kidney and the heart.

Gall bladder meridian (GB) Runs from the head to the tip of the little toe. Linked with headaches, colds and muscle pain.

Liver meridian (Liv) Runs from the big toes to the chest and regulates the flow of *chi*.

Governor vessel (GV) Runs from just above the anus to the upper lip. Linked with vitality.

Conception vessel (CV) Runs down the centre of the body, from the roof of the mouth. Linked with vitality and sexuality.

The importance of timing

Each meridian has a time of day when it is at its most active, and so is most easily stimulated.

Lung: 3–5am
Large intestine: 5–7am
Stomach: 7–9am
Spleen: 9–11am
Heart: 11am–1pm
Small intestine: 1–3pm
Bladder: 3–5pm
Kidneys: 5–7pm
Pericardium: 7–9pm
Triple energizer: 9–11pm
Gall bladder: 11pm–1am
Liver: 1–3am

▶

The meridians

The main meridians have many acupressure points, of which only those that are used in the massages are shown here. Those that lie on yin meridians are numbered from the lowest point, such as the spleen, which is numbered from the big toe, while those on yang meridians are numbered from the highest point, such as the stomach, which starts under the eye.

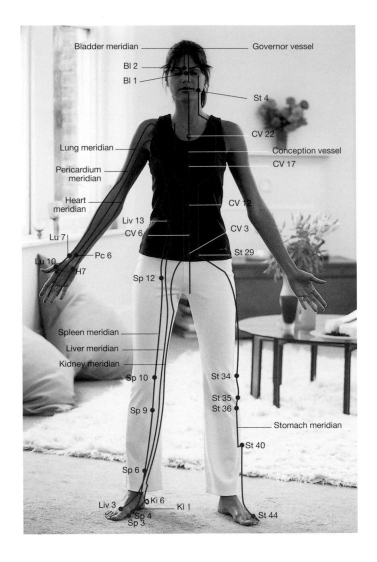

Bladder meridian
Governor vessel
Bl 2
Bl 1
St 4
CV 22
Lung meridian
Conception vessel
CV 17
Pericardium meridian
Heart meridian
CV 12
Liv 13
CV 3
CV 6
St 29
Lu 7
Pc 6
Lu 10
H7
Sp 12
Spleen meridian
Liver meridian
Kidney meridian
Sp 10
St 34
St 35
Sp 9
St 36
Stomach meridian
St 40
Sp 6
Liv 3
Ki 6
Ki 1
Sp 4
St 44
Sp 3

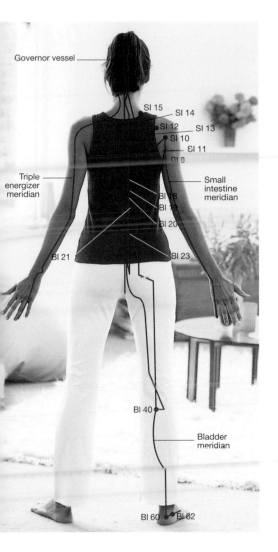

Governor vessel

SI 15
SI 14
SI 12
SI 13
SI 10
SI 11
SI 9

Triple
energizer
meridian

Small
intestine
meridian

Bl 18
Bl 19
Bl 20

Bl 21
Bl 23

Bl 40

Bladder
meridian

Bl 60
Bl 62

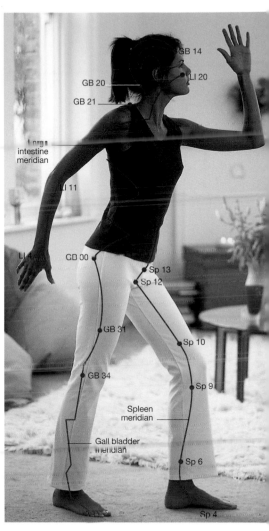

GB 14
GB 20
LI 20
GB 21

Large
intestine
meridian

LI 11

LI 4
GB 30
Sp 13
Sp 12

GB 31

Sp 10

GB 34
Sp 9

Spleen
meridian

Gall bladder
meridian

Sp 6

Sp 4

Head massage

One of the oldest known therapies, head massage, often known as Indian head massage, aids relaxation and boosts energy, while paying attention to key tension sites such as the face, head, scalp, neck and shoulders. It can also help improve concentration, reduce tension and stress, boost circulation, increase oxygen uptake in the body's cells and relieve the pain of headaches and eyestrain.

Head masssage is also used to stimulate the growth of hair and can combat hair loss caused by such factors as high blood pressure, poor circulation, disease and ageing. In India, this technique has been practised for nearly 4,000 years, and a head massage with natural oils is thought to nourish hair and promote circulation.

Techniques

A range of simple, basic techniques are used in head massage, which fall into the following main categories.

Gentle friction

These slow, rhythmic movements are warming, soothing and calming. They can be used on almost anybody at any time without using lubricants. Their slow rhythmic nature makes them comforting to the receiver and relaxing for the giver.

Smoothing

Can be used over the head, hair, face, neck, shoulders and back, warming the muscles at

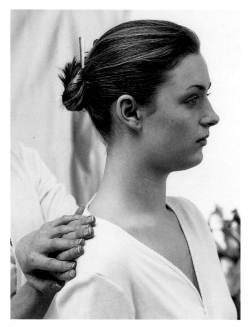

Smoothing

Interlacing

the beginning of a massage and relaxing them afterwards. Its stronger action towards the heart assists the return of venous blood, and its lighter application away from it removes energetic 'impurities'.

Interlacing

This is a slightly more powerful version of the smoothing technique. It involves placing the 'mother' hand (see box, below) on top of the 'working' one and interlacing the fingers to provide a broad platform with which to work on larger body areas, such as the back. The natural pattern of application is a small or large figure of eight.

Scrubbing

Less expansive and more localized than the smoothing and interlacing techniques, scrubbing allows you to work into the smaller contours of the body. Because of its more rapid application, it has a stronger localized warming effect.

The technique entails making a claw of your

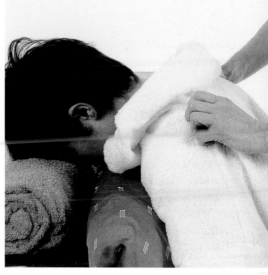

Scrubbing

working hand, then 'scrubbing' the flat of your nails, in small circular movements, over the muscle areas of the shoulders, back and upper arms. Scrubbing should be applied only up to the level of the recipient's preference/tolerance.

'Mother' and 'working' hands

When you are massaging, your less-dominant hand is simply used to maintain an energetic and comforting connection with the receiver. Known as the 'mother' hand, it is largely static and supportive, and is used to 'listen' for reactions to your treatments. The 'working' hand, whether left or right by preference, is the more active agent.

In the example shown, the mother hand provides support and stability to the forehead while the working hand gently elongates the neck.

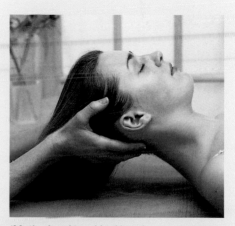

'Mother' and 'working' hands

▶

Stretching and aligning

These are gentle fine-tunings of postural alignment, to re-educate poor posture, so often the cause of chronic pain, muscular distress and common conditions such as headaches and depression. They can greatly ease tension from the neck and spine.

Traction

Using one of the gentle friction techniques, first warm and relax the muscles of the neck and shoulders. Sit or stand squarely behind the receiver, roughly half a head higher. Cradle their head in your hands, with your palms supporting the base of their skull and your fingers under the jawline. Take the weight of their head in your hands, lifting slightly as you bring your forearms between the shoulder blades and either side of the spine. Gently ease the head back using the forearms as both support and lever. Hold for two or three breaths, ease back to the central starting position and repeat slowly three times.

Tilting

Stand or sit to one side of or just behind the receiver. Place your working hand under their chin for support, with your opposite forearm resting lightly on the trapezius muscles, which run down the back of the neck along the shoulders. Initially place the mother hand on the other shoulder. As you slowly tilt the head back, bring the mother hand forearm round underneath the neck to support the movement. Gently ease the head backwards and forwards with the support of the working hand and forearm. Repeat the tilting movement three to six times.

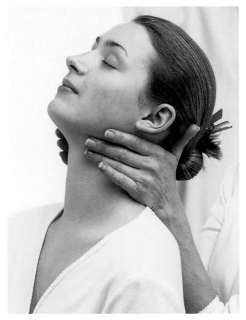

Traction

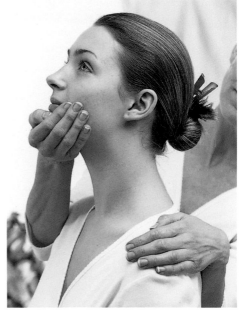

Tilting

Easing and comforting

Light and rhythmical, these movements are easy to learn and can be used at any time during a massage session. Although not a massage technique in itself, cradling is included because it provides a comforting and supportive end to a session.

Circling

Position your hands lightly on the shoulders on either side of the neck. Place the thumbs on the muscles on either side of the spine as far down as you can reach. Starting with an inward and upward circle, use the full pressure of your thumbs to make circling movements on the often-tight trapezius muscles between the shoulder blades. Start with large circles (right thumb clockwise, left thumb anticlockwise) on the area closest to the shoulder blade.

Piano walking

Imagine you are playing the piano on the trapezius and other soft muscle areas. The pressure you apply will depend on your own personal strength, how comfortable it is for your partner and your intuition of the moment. The technique, suitably modified in pressure, can also be used to great effect over the skull and along the neck. Pressure is applied from the tips of the fingers and should be attempted only if the nails are short enough not to indent the skin too much. Smooth at the end with some interlacing.

Cradling

This is a wonderful finishing touch or a step that can be used within a massage. Cradle the receiver's body close to yours and gently rock from side to side or round in small circles.

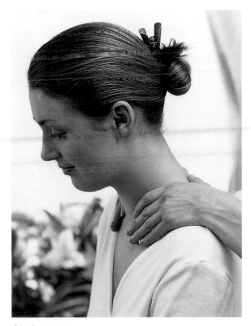

Circling

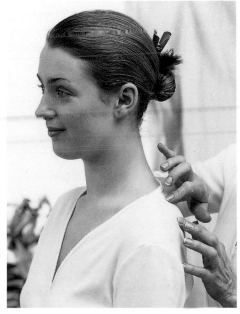

Piano walking

Thai massage

The roots of Thai massage lie in Buddhism. Massage and other healing arts were taught in the monasteries, and passed down through the generations. Today it is practised throughout Thailand, particularly in rural areas where access to hospitals is limited. Thai massage works by helping restore balance in the flow of energy throughout your body by stimulating energy lines and points. It works on both the superficial and deeper layers of muscles, ligaments, joints and connective tissues, and it touches all areas of the body including the nervous, digestive and respiratory systems. It can also increase flexibility, stretch and tone muscles, relieve many common ailments and help to achieve a general sense of wellbeing, vitality and relaxation.

How it works

Thai massage is a 'whole-body' strategy. While relaxation, for example, may be the initial goal, it will also improve suppleness and circulation, and lead to a more positive frame of mind.

The energy lines in Thai massage are called *sen* lines, which follow the form of the body and are connected to the entire body, mind and spirit. The energy that runs through the *sen* lines powers the physical, mental and emotional functions. When it is flowing smoothly and is balanced, we are free from illness. If the energy supply is deficient or when it is blocked, we may become unwell. Thai massage works on the body through applying pressure to stimulate energy flow.

Although the *sen* lines are reminiscent of the meridians, they should not be confused with them. While the meridians are associated with specific organs, and pressure is applied to

certain meridians in order to increase energy flow to a particular organ, the *sen* lines instead follow the form of the body and are connected to the entire body, mind and spirit.

Thai massage benefits both the giver and the receiver: both emerge from a session feeling more open, stretched, refreshed and balanced.

The *sen* lines
Inside leg

1 Starts above the ankle bone, travels along the underside of the shin bone, jumps across the knee to resurface one thumb-length down from the centre of the kneecap and continues straight up to the crease line at the groin.
2 Starts under the ankle bone, half way between 1 and 3, travels up the middle of the calf muscle, jumps across the knee, resurfacing

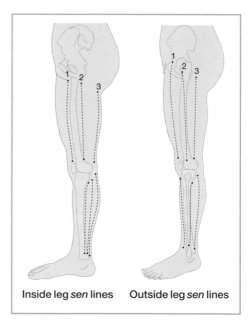

Inside leg *sen* lines   Outside leg *sen* lines

two thumb-lengths down from the centre of the kneecap, and continues straight up the middle of the inner thigh to the crease line at the groin, half way between 1 and 3.

3 Starts on the inner edge of the Achilles tendon behind the ankle, travels straight up the underside of the calf muscle and jumps over the knee to resurface three thumb-lengths down from the centre of the kneecap, ending at the start of the near-side buttock.

Outside leg

1 Starts on the front side of the ankle, runs up in the groove alongside the shin bone, jumps across the knee and resurfaces one thumb-length down from the centre of the kneecap and continues straight up to the crease line of the leg/hip.

2 Starts above the ankle bone, runs up the centre of the calf half way between 1 and 3, jumps across the knee, resurfaces two thumb-lengths down from the centre of the kneecap and continues up the centre of the outer thigh between 1 and 3 to the crease line at the hip.

3 Starts under the backside of the ankle bone, sitting on the Achilles tendon, runs up along the outside edge of the calf, jumps across the knee, resurfaces three thumb-lengths down from the centre of the kneecap and continues up the outside edge of the thigh to the crease line at the hip.

Front

1 Itha Starts at the navel, runs down the front of the left thigh, turns left at the knee, ascends the back of the left thigh, ascends the left side of the spine (in a laminar groove) and over the top of the head, finishing at the left nostril.

2 Pingala Takes the same course as Itha, but on the right side.

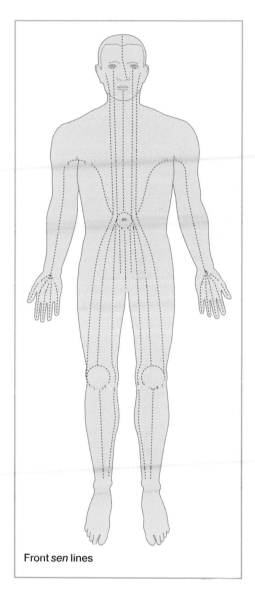

Front *sen* lines

3 Sumana Starts at the navel, runs straight up and inside the throat, finishing at the base of the tongue.

4 Kalatharee Starts at the navel and divides into four branches. Two branches descend through the groin and down the legs, ending at the toes. The other two branches ascend to the armpits, and run down the arms, stopping at the fingers.

5 Sahatsarangsi Starts at the navel, descends the inner left leg, turns at the ankle and runs back up the body, through the throat and finishes at the left eye.

6 Tawaree Takes the same course as Sahatsarangsi, but on the right side.

7 Lawusang Starts at the navel, runs up through the throat and stops at the left ear.

8 Ulanga Takes the same course as Lawusang, but on the right side.

9 Nantakawat Starts at the navel and divides into two branches:

Sukumang – stops at the anus;

Sikinee – stops at the urethra.

10 Kitcha Starts at the navel and descends to the sex organs:

Kitchana – clitoris;

Pittakun – penis.

Techniques

There are a number of techniques for working on the *sen* lines.

Palm press

This is used throughout and must be used before and after you work the *sen* lines to relax the limb you are working on. It prepares an area for deeper pressure work and relaxes the body between different procedures. The focus of contact is from the centre point of your palm as a 'warm beam of light'. Keep fingers relaxed and try not to apply pressure from the heel of your hands. Palm press is generally used in an alternate hand-rocking side-to-side motion.

For alternate palm press, keeping your own body relaxed and balanced, with the arms straight, lean your weight not too heavily onto one palm, then onto the other and back again, in a steady rocking motion. As you rock onto one hand, move the other up the limb, rock onto it, then bring your free hand up to follow it.

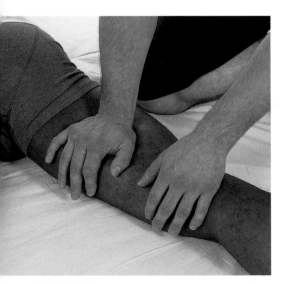

Palm press

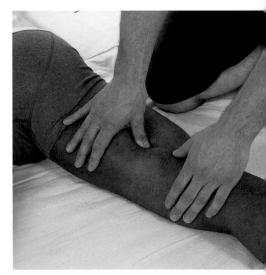

Thumb press

Thumb press

Pressure is applied by the thumb pad, never from the point or the tip. To ensure this, place the thumb flat against the point you are working on. The angle of delivery is always perpendicular. Apply enough pressure to be felt, but not enough to cause pain. Keep the rest of the hand relaxed, or tension will flow into the thumb. Do not use the thumb press directly on bones or tendons. Apply in the same way as the palm press, with a rocking motion.

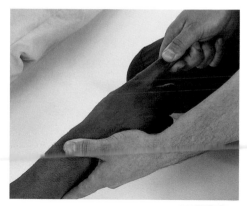

Slide stretch

Slide stretch

This is a slow pulling movement used on fingers and toes. Support the hand or foot you are working on with one hand. Grasp the finger or toe between the thumb and index finger of the other hand, squeeze firmly and simultaneously slide the fingers along the digit.

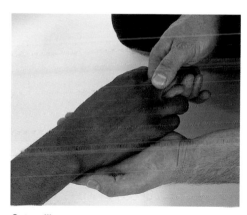

Caterpillar

This is generally applied to fingers and toes. Gently hold the digit between the thumb pad and the middle of your cupped index finger. Use alternate thumb and index finger actions, applying pressure away towards the toe or fingertip in a caterpillar-like movement.

Caterpillar

Thumb circles

This can be used all over parts of the body. Using the thumb press on bony areas such as the back of the hands or the top of the feet causes pain, which is why this more gentle circular movement of the thumbs is substituted. Your fingers should be relaxed yet supportive. Firmer pressure can be applied to the trapezius, which runs down the back of the neck and along the shoulders. Apply pressure through the thumb pad and circle in a clockwise direction away from the centre of the body area.

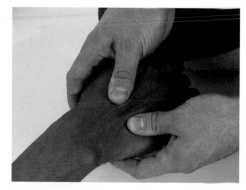

Thumb circles

Shiatsu

Shiatsu originated in Japan as a holistic therapy for treating the mind, body and spirit. Although it is now a popular 21st-century therapy, it is still closely related to its ancestral roots in ancient Oriental medicine. The healing art of shiatsu involves applying pressure to acupressure points (see pages 24–25), known in shiatsu as *tsubos*, and uses gentle manipulation techniques to rebalance the natural energy within the body so that the body can heal itself and maintain good health. The word shiatsu means 'finger pressure' in Japanese, although in fact other parts of the hand, as well as the elbows, knees and feet, are also used.

The symptoms that shiatsu can treat include back pain, headaches, whiplash injuries, neck stiffness, period pains, asthma and depression. Regular sessions can also help prevent the level of stress we experience in our daily lives building up to become a problem.

How it works

Shiatsu works on the body's energy system, which is based on the flow of *ki* or *chi*, a vital force of energy, using relatively few and very simple techniques to influence the muscles and circulation. For various reasons, *ki* may stop flowing freely, which then produces a bodily symptom. Shiatsu techniques improve the energy flow, as a result of which the symptoms will improve. The gentleness and simplicity of these movements belies the significance of the impact that they have on the underlying energies of the body. Different techniques are used to treat specific problems and relieve pain or to release energy blockages.

Techniques

The key to all shiatsu massage techniques is to channel your whole body weight through whatever 'tool' you are using – whether it be palms, thumbs, fingers, elbows, knees or feet – to apply pressure, which should come through the forward movement of your lower body. The idea is that rather than pressing your hands into the receiver, you lean and let your body weight do the work for you, applying a natural amount of pressure.

Palming

This is one of the most widely used shiatsu techniques and involves leaning your body weight into the open palm or heel of your hand, with your fingers relaxed but remaining in contact with the receiver, to apply a gentle yet firm pressure. This is a non-specific, comforting technique for restoring the free flow of *ki* and is best used on each part of the body as a prelude to the more precise pressure applied in the thumbing technique.

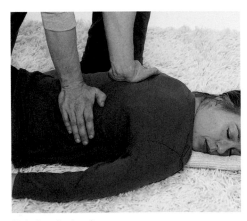

Palming the back

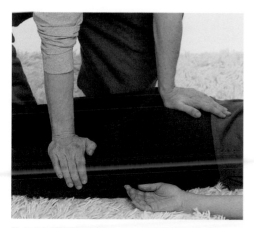

Palming the inner leg

Thumbing

This technique uses the outstretched thumb to apply specific, penetrating pressure, particularly to *tsubos*. It has a more stimulating effect than palming. There are two versions of thumbing: the stronger technique involves using the tip of the thumb, while the milder version uses the ball of the thumb in a more flattened position. Keep the fingers extended and in contact with the receiver to steady your thumb and to help support your weight.

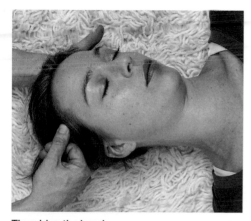

Thumbing the head

The major meridians

Ki flows around the body through an intricate network of channels, called meridians, the same as those used in acupressure (see pages 24–25). Each of the 12 primary meridians is linked to an organ, and most of the main *tsubos* – the points at which *ki* is more accessible and where it can be influenced through the application of pressure – are distributed along these meridians, which lie near to the surface.

Intersecting these meridians are another eight, more deeply lying, channels, which include the two channels that control all the others. One of these controlling channels is the 'governing vessel', a reservoir of yang, or masculine, energy that oversees the other yang channels (stomach, large and small intestines, bladder and gall bladder) and runs up the spine and over the head.

The other channel is the 'conception vessel', or 'directing vessel', which is its yin, or feminine, counterpart and oversees the yin channels (lung, spleen, heart, kidneys and liver), and which runs up the centre of the abdmomen and chest to the throat and mouth.

Yin and yang

According to most ancient Eastern medical texts, everything in the world, whether it is physical or immaterial, is composed of and affected by the forces of Yin and Yang – which can be defined as Darkness-Light, Passive-Active, Female-Male, Cold-Hot, Water-Fire, Open-Closed, Soft-Hard. When this natural balance in humans is disturbed by external forces such as injury, or internally by factors such as stress, shiatsu can be employed to readjust the flow of *ki* to restore health.

Ailments

In this section you will find a variety of fast and effective massage remedies, featuring the types of massage introduced in the previous section, for a wide range of commonly occurring ailments. Choose whichever individual therapy suits your circumstances or mood – they are not presented in any order of importance or designed to be performed as an overall sequence. And if you're really under pressure, there are 'quick fixes' on offer to bring rapid relief. Some massages are one-step techniques, while others require two or more steps and are numbered accordingly.

Mind and head

38–67

- Headache
- Migraine
- Stress
- Fatigue
- Insomnia
- Feeling down
- Eyestrain

- Sinusitis
- Earache
- Toothache
- Sore throat

Body

68–107

- Backache
- Stiff neck and shoulders
- Frozen shoulder
- Painful joints
- Tired feet
- Repetitive strain injury
- Tennis elbow
- Muscle cramps

- Poor circulation
- Digestive problems
- Stressed stomach
- Nausea/travel sickness
- Constipation

Female body

108–123

- PMT and menstrual pain
- Early pregnancy
- Mid-pregnancy
- Late pregnancy
- Menopause
- Cystitis

Headache

Most headaches are triggered by stress or bad posture, but they can also be caused by congestion, a raised temperature and viruses. Head massage can readjust the balance of pressures in the head, clearing sinuses, de-stressing neck and shoulder muscles and relieving eyestrain. The pain usually manifests itself at the base of the skull, in the temples and forehead, and at the top of the head.

Quick fixes

Use these techniques to quickly ease the discomfort of a headache:

- Lavender essential oil can bring instant relief when applied to tense areas. Put a few drops of lavender essential oil on your fingertips. Use a circular movement around the temples and along the forehead for a few minutes, working the oil well in to relieve any pain or energy blocks, until the pain or tension eases.

- To clear congestion, use your finger to apply firm pressure to the webbing between the thumb and index finger.

- Massaging the feet can encourage excess energy away from the head, relieving local pain felt there.

Head massage

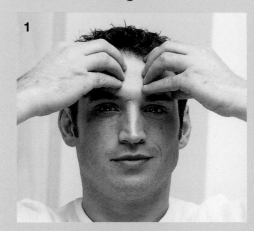

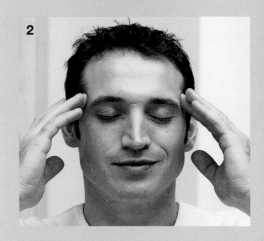

Tension headache
1 Place your fingertips on your forehead, applying a little pressure. Stroke outwards from the centre to the temples. Repeat three times.

2 Keeping your shoulders and elbows relaxed, place your middle fingers on the indentation of the temples and gently massage with small, circular movements. Repeat six times.

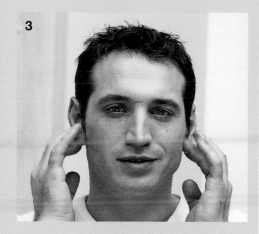

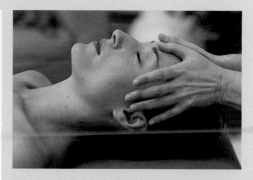

Headache at the front of the head

Gently circle your hands clockwise, without touching, about 6 cm (2.5 in) away from the temples to soothe. Use your fingers to make small, circular movements over the forehead to induce relaxation. Place both thumbs together in the centre of the forehead, just below the hairline. Work in a line up to the centre of the head, pressing and releasing the thumbs.

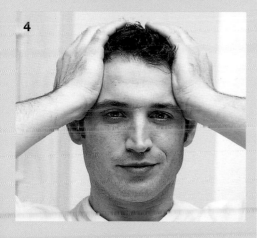

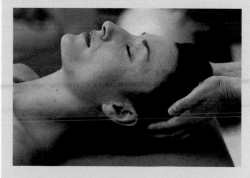

3 Using your middle fingers, massage down the side of the face to the hinge of the jaw, just below the earlobes. Circle around the area and repeat six times.

4 Fit the palms of your hands into the grooves of the temples. Squeeze gently with the heels of your hands and then make slow, wide circles six times in this area.

Headache at the back of the head

Gently circle your hands clockwise, without touching, about 6 cm (2.5 in) away from the base of the neck to the skull for relaxation. To improve circulation, apply firm pressure with your hands as you move them in a circular motion over the head.

▶

Reflexology

The brain and central nervous systems are centred in the big toe, so you need to work this area to treat headaches.

- To stimulate the brain, thumb- or finger-walk up the pad of the big toe several times, until you have covered the whole area.

- For a headache caused by sinuses, squeeze the sides and back of each toe.

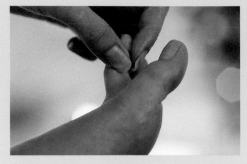

Treating a sinus headache

- For a headache caused by tiredness, ease it by pressing just below the big toenail. Then walk your index finger down the front and sides of the toe. Remember always to move in a direction away from your body.

- For a tension headache, slide diagonally down from the centre of the big toe pad to the corner of the pad beside the next toe. This is the occipital spot (see page 18), representing the bony ridge of the back of your skull.

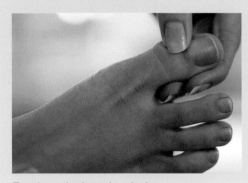

Treating a tiredness headache

Shiatsu

Applying pressure to points around the eye socket is particularly effective. In shiatsu, a headache is viewed as a sign of a blockage in the flow of *ki*, and therefore relates to the body's whole energy system. In this way, working on other areas of the body in addition, such as the arms, can bring lasting relief.

- Use your little finger to stimulate Bl 1 (see page 24), the point just above the inner corner of the eye. Apply the pressure inwards and upwards. Continue by working the other points around the eye sockets in the same way.

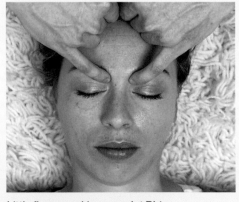

Little finger working on point Bl 1

Acupressure

Different parts of the head relate to different meridians and blockages. Since all the meridians pass through the neck, a neck massage often eases the problem wherever it started.

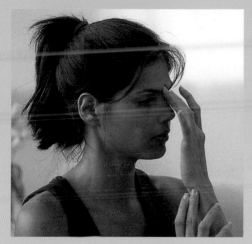

Massaging the 'third eye' point

- Concentrate on the hairline at the base of the skull. Also work on the trigger points (see page 22), gently moving the skin in circles, then stroking the energy down and away. Find the 'third eye' point, which lies in the centre of the forehead between the eyebrows or just above that point. Feel for a tiny natural dip

- You can also ease headaches by working on your hands and feet. For hands, start from the wrist below your little finger and run the opposite index finger up and down the sides of the fingers as if drawing an outline of your hand, ending at the bottom of the thumb. Pull each finger and thumb as if pulling a cap off it. Work your way around all the fingernails by pressing in with your fingernail to open the meridians. Massaging the foot can encourage excess energy away from the head, relieving local pain.

- With the receiver sitting cross-legged, with their back to you, use the palming technique to work down the small intestine meridian, from behind the shoulder joint along the back of the arm to the elbow, turning slightly onto the forearm, then down to the wrist and along the edge of the hand to the end of the little finger.

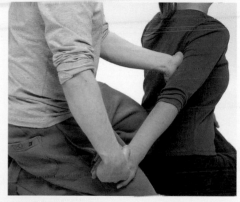

Palming the small intestine meridian

Migraine

Migraine is a severe headache lasting from two hours to two days, often accompanied by visual disturbances and nausea/vomiting. It is often triggered by food, so start by using reflexology techniques to work on areas that relate to the digestive system, then move on to the head and the spine – often the seat of tension that leads to headaches. You may also need to work on points for the relief of related symptoms, such as eyestrain or dizziness.

Quick fixes

Try to stop a migraine in its tracks as soon as you notice the onset:

- To induce relaxation, knead the base of the neck and the area across the top of the shoulders.
- Try to release pressure by using your thumb to gently press under the base of the skull.
- To help increase blood circulation, move your fingers gently over the scalp in a circular motion.

Reflexology

Toe area routine

1 The pituitary gland, controlling the hormone production of all other glands, is represented by a spot in the exact centre of the big toe pad (see page 18). Hold the foot in the supporting hand, with the fingers behind the big toe, and hook into the pituitary point with the thumb of the working hand, using four-finger leverage against the supporting hand.

2 After five seconds, use the opposite thumb to press into the hypothalamus reflex on top of the big toe, just above the pituitary.

3 Next, work the side of the big toe next to the second toe, to stimulate the neck muscles.

4 Move on to work the other side, down the inner edge of the foot, which relates to the vertebrae of the spine (see page 20).

Acupressure

Working several different areas of the body will help to relieve migraine.

- Find pain points halfway down the top of the hand, between the second and third, and the fourth and fifth hand bones. Lightly pull the fingers away from the hand.
- Work the back of the neck, GB 20 (see page 25), at the base of the skull.
- Massage the back beside the spine and above the waist, pushing gently outwards and downwards, to work on the bladder point Bl 20.

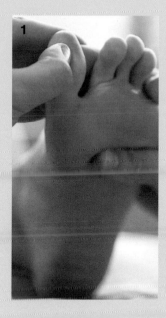
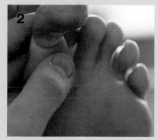
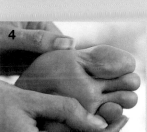
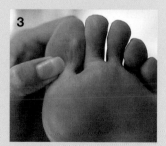
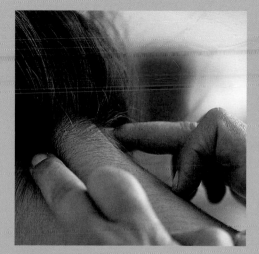
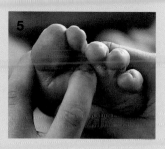

5 For the eyes (left eye on the left foot, right eye on the right foot), press into the fleshy area between and just below the bottom of the second and third toes, supporting with the other hand. Press and hold in this place for three to five seconds.

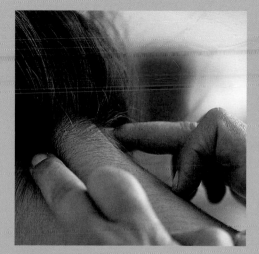

Working on point GB 20

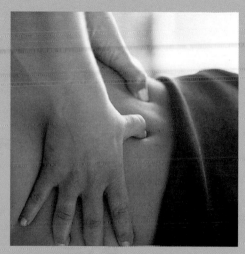

Working on the bladder point BI 20

Stress

Stress is a big factor in life today and it can lead to anxiety, lethargy, depression and loss of self-esteem. These have a negative effect on your health, showing up as muscular tension and headaches. If the stress that produces adverse symptoms is not handled properly, more serious illnesses may result. Regular massage will help reduce physical tension and naturally raise your endorphin levels, making you feel more positive.

Quick fixes

Try these simple measures to bring rapid relief from stress:

- Using your thumb tips, apply small, gentle, rhythmic strokes running up the middle of the forehead.
- Work up and down the muscles on either side of the spine in the shoulder area, applying firm pressure with your thumbs, then making circular movements and squeezing the muscles.
- Using your fingertips, apply gentle rhythmic strokes down each leg in turn, from the hip to the toe.

Head massage

Anxiety release

1 Position yourself behind the receiver's head and, leaning forward, place the fingers of both hands on the chin. With your finger pads rotating in small circles, move along very slowly around the jawline to just in front of the earlobes.

2 Place your thumbs together and flat to the surface at the centre of the forehead, holding the sides of the head. Glide each thumb outwards to the temples, lift off and return to the centre. Repeat several times, moving up over the whole of the forehead to the hairline.

Acupressure

To combat the negative effects of stress, and to release tension and anxiety:

- Work on points Liv 3 (between the big and second toes, two finger-widths up the foot from the join between the toes), LI 4 and H 7 on the hand and wrist (see pages 24–25).

- Breathe deeply while touching the 'sea of energy', CV 6, two finger-widths below the navel, or while gently massaging the heart point, CV 17.

- Rub the stomach both clockwise and anticlockwise, or massage the inside border of the shoulder.

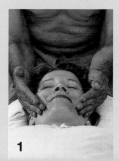

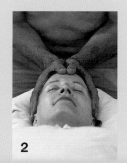

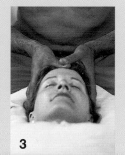

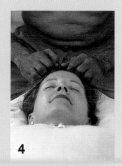

1   **2**   **3**   **4**

3 Place your thumbs on top of each other at the centre of the forehead near the hairline, then exert pressure, hold for a few seconds and release. Repeat, moving up over the head to the centre.

4 Draw the splayed fingers of both hands very slowly through the receiver's hair in a combing action, moving one hand and then the other in a continuous, rhythmic motion.

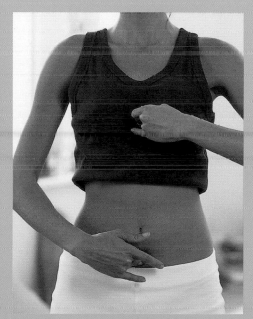

Massaging the 'sea of energy' and the heart point

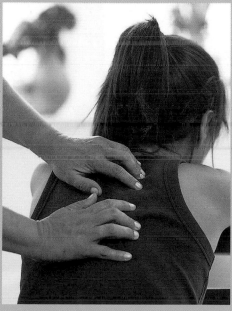

Massaging along the inside edge of the shoulder blade

Reflexology

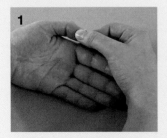

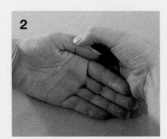

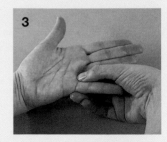

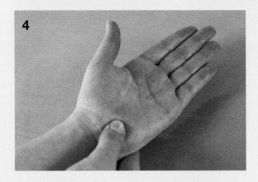

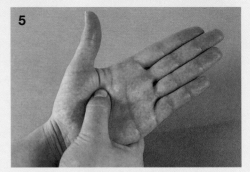

Stress-relieving hand routine

1 Support your thumb on the fingers of one hand. Use your working thumb to stimulate the outside edge of the thumb. Take deep breaths while you stimulate with small circles.

2 Cradle one hand in the other. Use your working thumb to thumb-walk along the bone of the thumb from the first to the second joint. Continue to walk along the bone from the second joint to the base of the hand.

3 Place your working thumb halfway down the palm of your hand between zones 4 and 5 (see page 17). Apply pressure and thumb-walk towards the base of the fingers and between the bones. Continue in this manner between zones 3 and 4 and zones 2 and 3.

4 Place your working thumb at the base of zone 4 just above your wrist. Turn your thumbnail so that it faces up to the ring finger. Walk up zone 4 until halfway up the hand. Push down and stimulate before turning to walk across the hand, ending up between the webbing between finger and thumb.

5 Support one hand in the other. Place your working thumb in the webbing just above the thumb muscle halfway down the hand. Use your thumb to hook into the webbing and apply pressure.

Thai massage

Shoulder tension release

1 Adopt a half-kneeling stance directly behind the receiver. Gently knead the trapezius muscles, which run down the back of the neck and along the shoulders, with the heel of alternate hands.

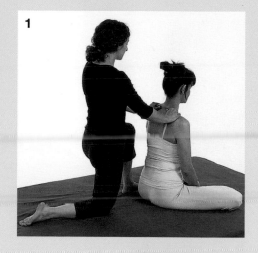

2 Massage the trapezius with your thumbs, using a circular squeezing motion. Take care that your fingers do not pinch the front of the receiver's shoulders.

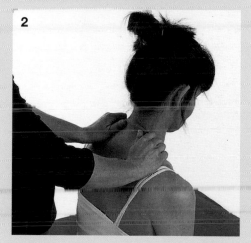

Correct posture

The receiver's back must be aligned as straight as possible, but still be relaxed, before you start. If the receiver is unable to sit cross-legged, this exercise can be adapted so that they can sit on a stool or sit facing the back of a dining chair.

Fatigue

If your busy lifestyle leaves you feeling routinely tired and a little rundown, think about how you can reduce your workload and make time for some form of enjoyable relaxation and a regular massage session to reinvigorate you. If, however, you constantly suffer from tiredness, in spite of not having done very much, this may be caused by depression, thyroid malfunction or a number of medical conditions, so consult your medical adviser.

Quick fixes

When energy is flagging, try the following reflexology treatment, or the simple palm press below:

- Thumb-walk down the spine area, which corresponds to the bony ridge of the hand from the side of the thumb down to the wrist (see page 21).

- Sit with your feet flat on the floor, pressing one palm on the base of your spine and the other palm just below your navel. Imagine you are breathing out fatigue, and breathing in a golden light that spreads energy throughout your body.

Reflexology

This form of therapy is as beneficial for the mind as the body, and when we experience fatigue, it is often mental as well as physical. These massages will help reinvigorate both mind and body.

- Start by focusing on the brain and the central nervous system, by working the big toe and the other toes, and including the spine reflex, which runs down the inside edge of the foot, from the big toe (see page 20).

- Work on the endocrine system (see page 20). Then focus on the adrenal glands by pressing and holding firmly on the kidney area and, with your other thumb pointing down the foot, quickly pressing into the adrenal point while releasing pressure on the kidneys (see page 18). Next work on the liver, located below the diaphragm, by hooking and applying firm pressure towards the fifth toe, then the thymus gland and the pituitary.

- Moving away from the feet, try tapping the breastbone, just below the collarbones, to stimulate the thymus.

Blocked energy

To help get energy moving around the body, work alternately on the hands and feet in the same session. You may find that there is very little reflex action in a tired person. The muscle tissue may feel slack, the hands and feet may feel cold and there may be a general feeling of emptiness or energy depletion in parts of the foot.

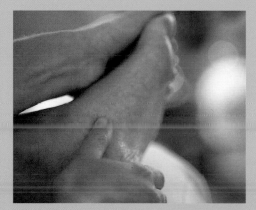

Working on the spine reflex

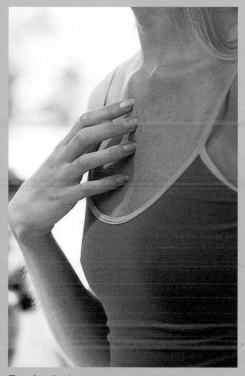

Tapping the breastbone can stimulate the thymus gland

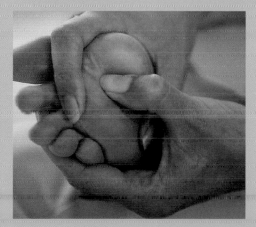

Working on the thymus gland in the foot

Head massage

To re-energize your body, try the following technique based on Joseph Corvo's 'zone therapy', which aims to unblock and rebalance your vital energies. Massaging this area, which is associated with the lungs, will improve your supply of oxygen, helping to give you a lift.

- Find the muscle running down the length of the side of your mouth. Then, using a rotating motion, press inwards and upwards as hard as you can bear for 30 seconds.

Insomnia

Insomnia is a side-effect of stress and is usually linked with anxiety about something in our lives. Massage promotes sleep naturally, and gentle, rhythmic strokes are particularly effective, as is a facial routine. The ideal time to massage is just before bedtime. Try to empty your mind of worries before you go to bed, and establish a calming routine every night.

Quick fixes

Use these two easy techniques to reduce tension and induce relaxation:

- Use the Western massage kneading technique to massage the whole shoulder and upper back area.

- Apply firm pressure to the soles of the feet with your thumbs, then apply gentle rhythmic strokes, working down from the heel to the toe.

Reflexology

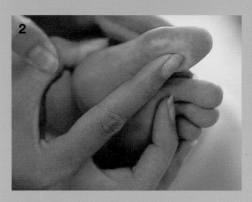

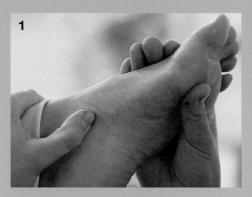

Relieving tension and rebalancing biorhythms

1 First work on the brain and central nervous system in the toes (see page 18), then the entire spine, from the neck at the side of the big toe to the coccyx at the corner of the heel bone, to relieve the underlying tension that frequently disturbs sleep (see page 20).

2 Next work on the pineal gland, which helps to balance the biorhythms. Then work on the pituitary gland to regulate hormones, and the adrenal glands, solar plexus and diaphragm to reduce anxiety.

Acupressure

The underlying cause of sleeplessness has a bearing on the specific treatment required, but the following will help in general to promote sound sleep.

- Massage the 'third eye' point between the eyebrows. Working on the heart meridian, using H 7 on the outer edge of the front of the wrist (see page 24), also has a calming effect on the mind.

- Alternatively, rub the insides and outsides of your heels to work on Ki 6, also known as 'close eyes', and Bl 62 (see page 25), or 'calm sleep'.

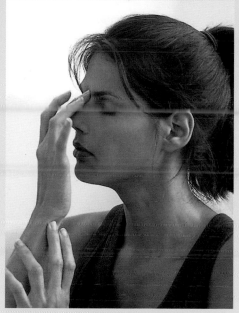

Working on the 'third eye' point and H 7

'Sweet dreams' oil

An essential oil such as lavender can be used to enhance the benefits of a sleep-inducing massage. The following mixture is especially effective in helping you to unwind: 12 drops of lavender, 8 drops of neroli and 5 drops of rose essential oils. Mix together and store in a glass bottle. For one massage session, mix half the mixture with 25 ml (1 fl oz) of almond, grapeseed or any other cold-pressed vegetable oil. For a really relaxing effect, massage it into the scalp, wrap your head in a towel and leave overnight.

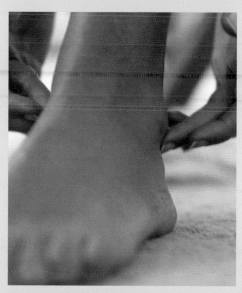

Working on Bl 62, 'calm sleep'

▶

Western massage

Self-massage for sleep

1 You can use the bedtime massage oil on page 51 to enhance the effects of this routine. Rest your three central fingers of each hand on each eyebrow. Close your eyes lightly and remain in that position for a moment, taking a few deep breaths.

2 Place the middle finger of each hand either side of, and immediately above, the bridge of your nose, between your eyebrows. Now, following the line of the brows, make small circles with your fingers along the length of your brows as far as your temples. When you reach your temples, hold your fingers over them for a moment with a slightly increased pressure. Return to the centre of the forehead, this time with your fingers placed slightly higher, and trace another line out towards your temples in the same way.

3 Continue to repeat Step 2, each time moving your fingers up slightly more until they are following the hairline. Continue following the hairline all the way round to the nape of your neck. Repeat several times.

4 Make the same circular movements from the neck hairline down your neck, with your fingers on either side of your spine. Do not place them on the spine itself.

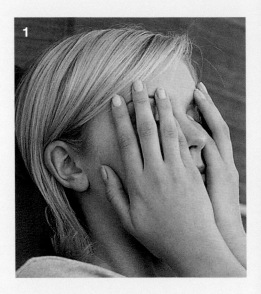

5 Use the same movements from the centre of your forehead back across your scalp to the nape of your neck. You may want to use two or three fingers here and make the movement cover a larger area. Finally, using your whole hands, cover the whole of your head, as if you were kneading your scalp.

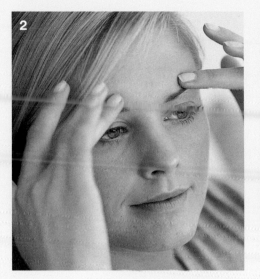

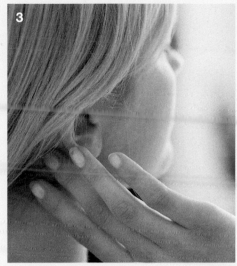

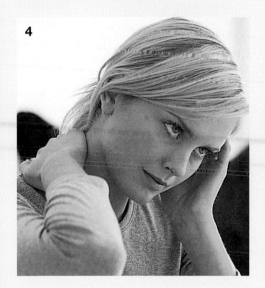

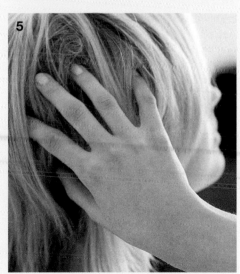

Feeling down

State of mind is closely associated with physical wellbeing. Negative emotions can manifest themselves in the body as disease if not corrected. Massage can help you cope with difficult situations and provide the quiet time necessary for giving you renewed mental energy and a positive outlook.

Quick fixes

For low spirits or mental stress, these quick techniques will help calm the nerves and lift the spirit:

- Place both hands on the head and very slowly make small circles into and over the scalp.

- Using your fingertips, make small circles up the centre of the forehead to the crown.

- Using your fingertips, make large circles over the upper back.

Reflexology

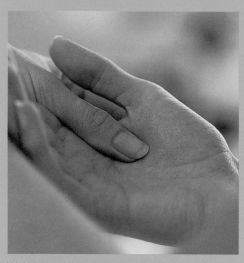

Working on the adrenals

It is important not to let low moods take hold, because they may develop into a prolonged depressive state of mind. Try this multifaceted mood-lifting hand therapy.

- Start with the brain and central nervous system, centred on the thumbs, then work on the kidneys – believed to be the site of suppressed tears – the adrenals (shown above) to lift exhaustion, the neck to relieve tension and the solar plexus to increase energy (see page 20).

- Work on the ileocaecal valve to stimulate the digestive system, which often becomes sluggish when you are depressed.

Acupressure

Follow this simple routine to rebalance your confused emotions.

- Work on the spleen meridian, which runs upwards from the big toe to the armpits, to 'earth' yourself (see page 25).

- Rub up and down the fleshy sides of the lower legs from the knee to the ankle, inside and outside, to stimulate Sp 4–10 and St 40.

- Lu 7 and Lu 10 are good points for releasing stagnation, allowing blocked energy to move and freeing repressed emotions.

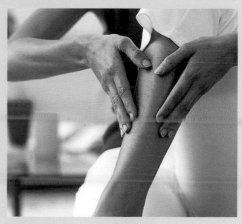

Stimulating Sp 4–10 and St 40

Thai massage

Emotional release

1 Move to a half-kneeling stance over the receiver, at waist level. Placing hand on hand, and using your middle fingers, circle with your fingers up the whole length of the breastbone. Open your hands, move to the collarbone and finger circle from the centre out and back along its lower edge, using both hands simultaneously.

2 Now work the spaces between the ribs (intercostals) in the same way, moving from the inside to the outside, then lowering to the next rib space. Return back up via the breastbone (excluding the breast area if you are working on a woman).

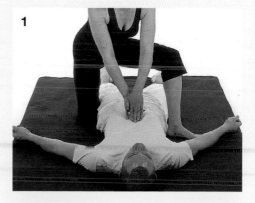

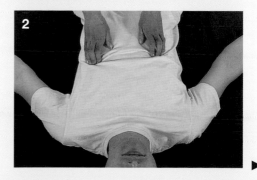

▶

Reflexology

Emotional pick-me-up

1 Support the fingers of one hand in the other and, using your working thumb, walk from the tip to the base or the base to the tip of one finger. Continue in this manner until you have worked all the fingers. Stimulate with tiny circles at each step.

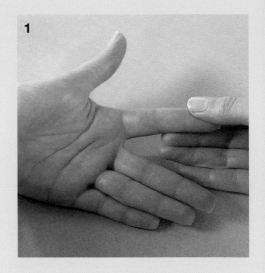

2 Place your working thumb a third of the way down the palm of your other hand and use the butterfly technique to walk across the hand from one side to the other.

3 Cradle your thumb in your fingers and use your working thumb to walk along the bone of the thumb from the first to the second joint. Make seven small steps along the bone, to represent the seven vertebrae in the neck. Stimulate with small circles at each step.

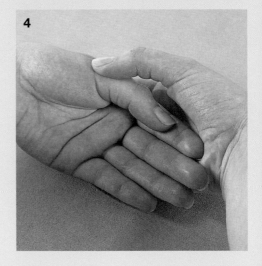

4 Cradle one hand in the other and use your working thumb to walk along the bone, starting at the base of the thumb. Make 12 small steps along the bone to the edge of the wrist. Continue along the bone to the base of the hand.

5 Support your thumb on the fingers of one hand and use your working thumb to stimulate the inside edge of the centre of your thumb. Take deep breaths while you stimulate with small circles.

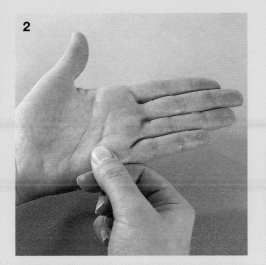

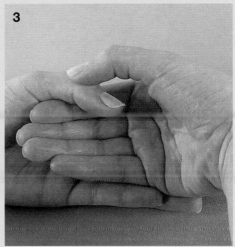

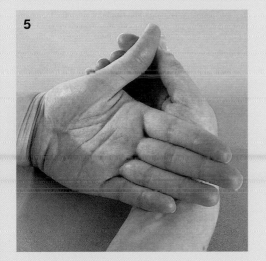

Regaining control

Gentle hand reflexology can help people cope with difficult situations that seem out of control. It provides a safe way of calming the emotions and has no unpleasant side-effects. A reflexology session will allow the quiet time necessary for letting new ideas generate, providing renewed mental energy and a positive outlook on life.

Eyestrain

In this modern world of computer screens, electronic media and bright lights, it is all too common to suffer from aching eyes or discomfort in or around the eyes. Eyestrain can also cause blurred vision, headaches and even migraines. Simple massage techniques can remedy the problem quickly and easily.

Quick fixes

For rapid relief from eye fatigue, try the following massages:

- Warm your hands by rubbing them together. Lightly place your cupped hands over the eyes. Maintain this position for a few minutes.
- Use your fingertips to apply firm pressure along the ridge of the lower eye socket.

Western massage

Treatment for tired eyes

1 Sit with your elbows on a firm surface. Place your fingers on the top of your head, rest your eyes into the heels of your hand and relax your whole body, letting your hands take the weight. Hold this position for 20 seconds, then release. Repeat four times.

2 Move the heels of your hands to rest on your eyebrows. Take a deep breath, and on the out breath, glide your hands from the inner ends of your eyebrows outwards and pull off at the side of the head, smoothing the entire browline. Repeat four times.

3 Move back to the inner ends of the eyebrows and place the pads of your thumbs underneath the inner edge with a level soft pressure that you are comfortable with. Hold for ten seconds and release. Repeat four times.

4 Place the middle two fingers of each hand on your temples and, using the pressure from your fingers as support, release your head and neck. Take a deep breath, and on the out breath, very slowly rotate your fingers clockwise. Repeat four times.

Acupressure

The acupressure points that help relieve eyestrain lie on the bladder meridian and the gall bladder meridian (see pages 24–25).

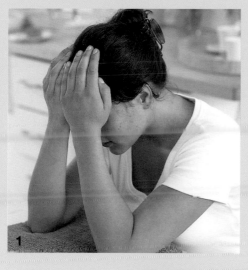

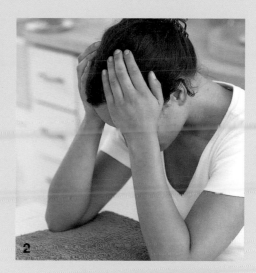

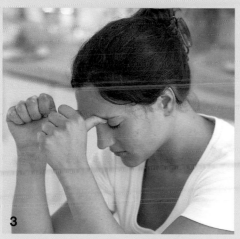

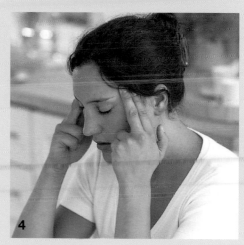

- Work on Bl 1, in the eye socket beside the inner edge of the eye.

- Target point GB 14, halfway up the forehead from the middle of each eyebrow.

- Pinch the bridge of the nose, just below the end of the eyebrow, at Bl 2.

Sinusitis

Self-massage, where you can regulate the pressure according to the severity of the condition, is effective in preventing congestion and relieving sinusitis. The sinuses are hollow, air-filled cavities that drain into the nose. Congestion or inflammation of the sinuses results in a heavy, blocked-up feeling accompanied by tension, and sometimes fever and a loss of the sense of smell.

Quick fixes

These measures will help bring you some swift comfort from the congestion and pain:

- Place your middle fingers on either side of your nose, breathe in and, on the out breath, glide your fingers down the sides of your nose to the nostrils and on to the cheeks, following the natural curve. Repeat. Palpate the areas at the beginning and end of the movement to help drain the sinuses.

- Apply firm pressure upwards along the centre line of the forehead to help soothe away tension.

Reflexology

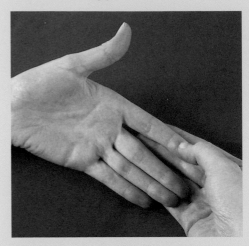

Working the sinuses reflex

Use this hand reflexology technique to work on the sinuses reflex in order to ease pressure and aid drainage (see page 20).

- Support the fingers of one hand in the other. Using your working thumb, walk from the tip to the base, or the base to the tip, of the index finger. Continue in this manner until you have worked all the fingers. Stimulate with tiny circles at each step.

Acupressure

This therapy offers a couple of easy techniques to help in the treatment of sinusitis.

• Run your fingers down the side of the nose and press into the wing at the bottom outer edge of the nostril, at point LI 20 at the end of the large intestine meridian (see page 25).

• On the base of your skull at the back, two points (GB 20) lie about four finger-widths apart, beside the top of the spine – nod your head to feel the two big muscles, then press in at the outside of them at the hairline.

Thai massage

This relaxing massage is good for draining sinuses and for easing throbbing headaches caused by the congestion.

• Lightly place your fingers around the receiver's jawline. Using both hands, simultaneously apply thumb presses. Follow the lines of the points as shown in the diagram below, starting at the chin and working up the face.

• Moving up, continue following other lines on the face with points around the eyes, finishing at the temples. Gently apply thumb circles at the end of each line.

• Finish with gentle strokes over the face and head in the direction of the neck to the forehead. Follow by gentle strokes of the hair.

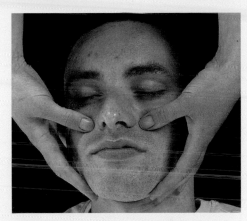

Applying thumb presses to the sinus area

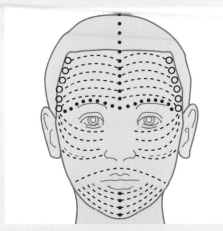

Facial lines and points used in Thai massage

Earache

The middle ear is the most common site in which infection can arise. This can lead to intense pain and raised temperature, while the inner ear can be affected by the spread of such infection. The outer ear can also suffer a bacterial or fungal infection. Massage techniques can help with the elimination of toxins, making the usual routes for the removal of toxins clearer, thus relieving the ears of this task.

Quick fix

You can perform this simple technique any time anywhere to bring quick relief from pain in the ear:

- Ease the head slightly to one side. Gently smooth up the crease behind one ear from the lobe to the top using the tips of your fingers. Repeat three times. Ease the head over and repeat behind the other ear.

Head massage

Try these simple facial massage techniques to help ease earache.

- Ease the head slightly to one side. Gently run the length of your index finger back and forth several times in the 'V' formed by the top part of the ear and the head. Ease the head over to the opposite side and repeat.

- Cup the jaw and firmly pinch the flesh of the chin between index fingers and thumbs. Firmly smooth along the jawline, finishing with six small circular movements in the 'hinge' just below the earlobes. Continue making circles with the index fingers to work the area, resting the thumbs lightly on the temples.

Reflexology

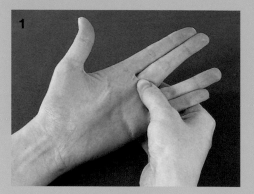

1

Ear reflexes routine

1 To work on the eustachian tube reflex (see page 20), support one hand in the other and place your working thumb between the middle and ring fingers. Apply pressure and stimulate with small circles.

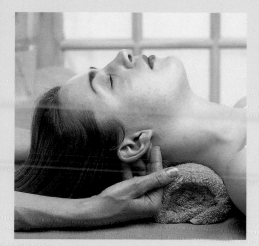

Working behind the ear

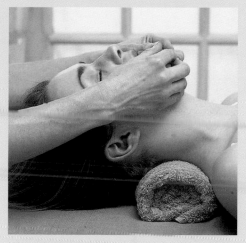

Working on the jawline

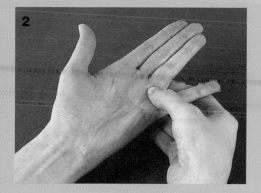

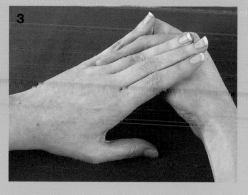

2 To work on the outer ear reflex, support one hand in the other and place your working thumb between the ring and little fingers. Apply pressure, tear towards the joint at the base of the little finger and stimulate with small circles.

3 To work on the inner ear reflex, turn the hand palm downwards, then place your working index finger and thumb on the joint at the base of the ring finger. Apply pressure and make small circles to stimulate.

Toothache

Most toothache is the result of tooth decay or gum disease, neuralgia, an abscess or sinusitis. Sometimes it can be brought on by eating something that irritates an exposed nerve. Massage techniques can help – for example, reflexology can be used to stimulate the points on the hands and feet corresponding to the teeth.

Quick fixes

For relief from toothache, try either or both of these measures:

- Give each hand an all-over massage, as there are several points on the hands that are beneficial for toothache.

- Gently massage the gum with some oil of cloves or whisky on your fingertip, as this will quickly numb the pain.

Acupressure

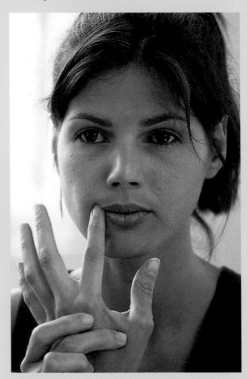

Stimulating St 4

Applying pressure to acupressure points can help alleviate the discomfort of toothache.

- Point LI 4, between the finger and thumb (not to be used during pregnancy) (see page 25), and St 4, at the corner of the mouth when the mouth is at rest (see page 24), are both good for relaxing the facial muscles to help ease cases of toothache.

Reflexology

There are two alternative approaches for treating toothache, the first probably being the most convenient.

- Working on the hands, start with finger- and thumb-walking, then thumb-walking or pressing and rotating along the first joint of the thumb, which corresponds to the jaw.

- Working on the feet, thumb-walk or press and rotate along the jawline points, located on the first joint of the big toe.

- To help ease pain coming from one or more teeth or from the gums, felt as a dull throb or as a sharp twinge, work on the teeth reflex as follows. Supporting your thumb, use your working index finger and thumb to walk between your thumbnail and the first joint, using the bird's beak technique.

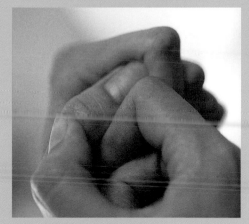

Stimulating the jaw reflex

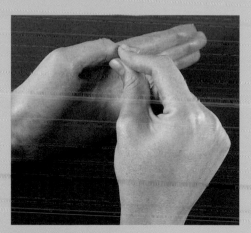

Working the teeth reflex

Sore throat

A sore throat is an inflammation of the pharynx, and is also known as pharyngitis. It often comes hand in hand with a cold, earache or flu, and clears up as soon as the worst of the illness passes. Sore throats are usually caused either by a virus or bacteria. Massage can help relieve symptoms and discomfort, particularly acupressure and reflexology techniques, which are also quick and easy to deliver.

Quick fixes

These two alternative thumb treatments will help soothe a painful throat:

- Holding the base of the thumb in one hand, work along both edges up towards the nail, squeezing as you go.

- Locate point Lu 10, two finger-widths up from the wrist, right on the edge of the thumb bone, and apply firm pressure with the thumb (see page 24).

Reflexology

Hand therapy for back of mouth and nose

1 To work on the head reflex, cup one thumb in your other hand and use your working thumb to walk down from the tip to the base of the thumb. Continue in this manner until you have covered the area. Stimulate with tiny circles at each step.

2 To work on the throat reflex, place your working thumb on the hiatus hernia point, and walk up between the bones to the bases of the index and middle fingers. Continue in this way, stimulating with small circles at each step.

3 To work on the lungs reflex, place your working thumb halfway down the palm of the hand between zones 5 and 4 (see page 17). Thumb-walk towards the base of the fingers and between the bones. Continue in this manner between zones 4 and 3 and zones 3 and 2.

4 To work on the kidney/adrenal reflex, support one hand with the other and place your working thumb in the webbing between the thumb and index finger just above the thumb muscle halfway down the hand. Use your thumb to hook into the webbing and apply pressure.

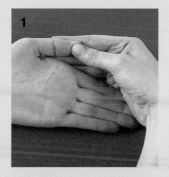

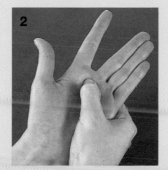

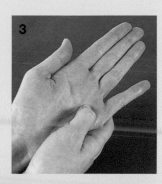

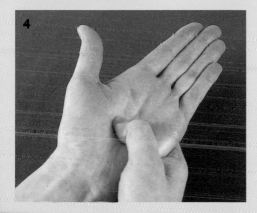

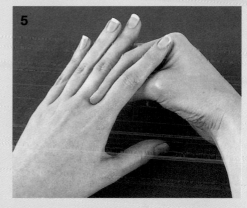

5 To work on the lymphatics reflex, place one hand palm downwards and place your working index finger and thumb between the bases of the index and middle fingers. Apply pressure and, using the bird's beak technique (see page 16), take tiny steps towards the wrist. Continue between zones 3 and 4 and 4 and 5.

Acupressure

Point CV 22, on the conception vessel, which runs down the centre of the body from the roof of the mouth (see page 24), can help relieve both sore throats and any accompanying phlegm or tightness in the chest.

- Work on this point, which is situated between the collarbones in the so-called 'salt cellar' – the dip between the collarbones.

Backache

Back pain accounts for more lost working days than any other complaint. The back is vulnerable because it is our main supportive structure and it stores enormous amounts of tension in the large muscles that cover the area. Massage techniques can be highly effective in releasing tension and relieving pain. But if back pain is persistent and has no obvious cause, consult your health adviser.

Quick fixes

Here are two simple ways to ease back pain, one for you and one for a partner:

- Using the flat of your hand, apply quick, light strokes away from the spine, to gently stretch out the muscles.

- Lie down on a couple of soft but firm juggling balls, one of them each side of the spine. Shift position to move them up and down the spine. If your back is very stiff or you have a back condition, check with your doctor before attempting this.

Western massage

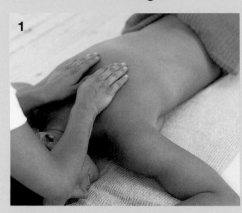

Whole back routine

1 Using the effleurage stroke, work on either side of the spine, gliding your hands downwards to the lower back. If you are working on the floor, you have to rise up on your knees in order to drop your weight behind the stroke as you stretch forwards towards the lower back area.

2 At the lower back, glide your hands outwards in opposite directions to the sides of the torso and then bring them up the sides with a slight pull, ending level with the armpits.

3 Bring your hands inwards towards the spine, gliding over the tops of the shoulder blades. At this stage, you can either repeat Steps 1–3 four or five times or continue with the sequence.

Acupressure

Work on the trigger points that correspond to where the pain is occurring (see page 22). In addition, try working on the following acupressure points:

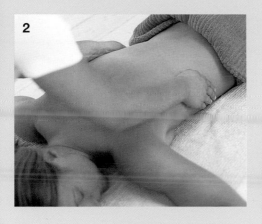

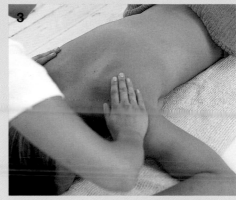

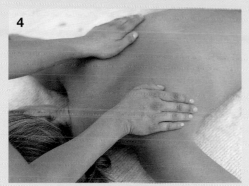

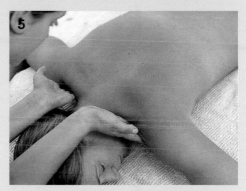

4 At the shoulder blades, turn your hands outwards and bring them over the top of the shoulders, so that the flats of your hands are now turned upwards, with the fingers resting on the front of the shoulders.

5 Scoop your hands inwards towards the neck. Repeat Steps 1–5 three or four times. On the final stroke, you may wish to bring your hands up the neck, finishing at the hairline.

- Put your thumbs on the hip bones, stretch your little fingers around the back and find the spot where your middle fingers end. This is GB 30 (see page 25).

- For sciatica, work on point GB 31 – mid-thigh on the outside of the leg – as well as Bl 40, behind the knee in the middle.

▶

Reflexology

The area that corresponds to the spine on your hand runs down the edge of the thumb to just above the wrist.

- To work the spine, finger- or thumb-walk all the way down the bony ridge (see page 21).

- To ease tired back muscles, use your four fingers and knead or walk horizontally across the bony ridge, searching for any sensitive areas. Finish with soothing massage strokes down the hand, covering the spinal reflexes.

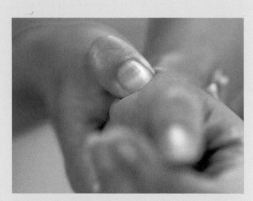

Thumb-walking along the spine

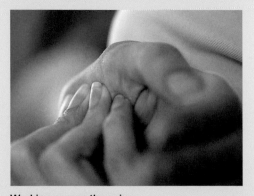

Working across the spine

Thai massage

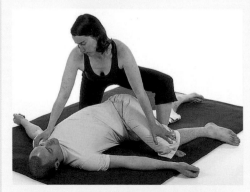

Lowering the leg as the lower back opens up

Follow this routine to release the lower back, mid-lumbar and thoracic spine.

- In a half-kneeling position, move your body around to face the receiver, very slowly bringing one leg across the body so that the thigh lies at a right angle to the torso.

- Place one hand on the upper knee and the other on the shoulder. Ask the receiver to breathe in, and on the out breath, tell them to relax. Allow the leg to lower itself as the lower back opens up.

- On each out breath, the receiver relaxes the leg a little more, allowing it to fall closer to the floor. Repeat on the other side.

Shiatsu
Bladder meridian massage

1 Position yourself at right angles to the receiver. Use the palming technique to work down the main bladder merdian, which runs parallel with the spine from the base of the skull to the sacrum, the triangular bone at the base of the spine (see page 25). Using one hand on the back or shoulder as a support, work down one side of the spine then the other.

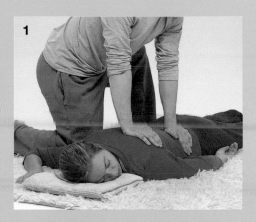

2 Work down the meridian, again on one side of the spine at a time, applying pressure with your elbows, gradually shifting your body weight forwards on to them. Draw back a little to move your elbows along the meridian. Stay in the same position to work the other side.

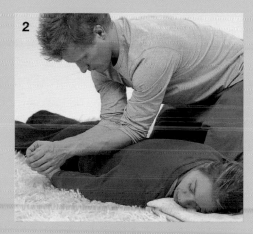

3 Change position and kneel beside the receiver's thighs. Find the sacrum and feel for two vertical rows of four hollows on either side. Apply pressure from both thumbs at once to the first pair of points, then repeat with the remaining three pairs.

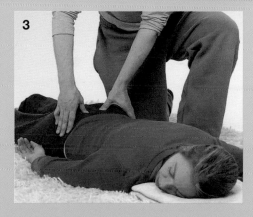

Stiff neck and shoulders

After a long day at work, tension can appear in the muscles of the shoulders and neck. This area is often the weakest part of the body and is also where most tension is stored. Lack of exercise and a sedentary lifestyle aggravate the problem. Aching shoulders are almost always caused by strain, and can often be relieved by improving your posture. Massage can be used to help muscles relax.

Quick fixes

Try this simple head massage to melt away tension in the neck, and the following acupressure technique to ease aching shoulders:

- Cradle the back of your head in your hands and circle your thumbs around the soft fleshy area at the base of the skull. Work methodically around the area to your own level of comfort.

- Gently press GB 21 on top of the shoulder, in the middle of the slope between the shoulder and neck, while you breathe out and visualize the pain leaving the spot (see page 25).

Reflexology

Shoulder ache relief

1 Knead and massage your way across both the top and the sole of the foot, about 2.5 cm (1 in) from the toes.

2 Pinch, press and gently hold for a count of five on the shoulder point located on the foot between the bases of the fourth and fifth toes (see page 19).

3 Repeat Step 2 on the shoulder reflex on the hand between the bases of the fourth and fifth fingers (see page 20).

Thai Massage

Tension release for neck

1 Half-kneel behind the receiver, who should be sitting upright. Ask them to lower their head a little.

2 Clasp your hands and warm the receiver's neck by squeezing the heels of your hands firmly together and working them up and down the neck.

3 Keep your hands clasped in the same position and lift your elbows. Place your thumbs on the receiver's neck in the laminar grooves on either side of the spine. Starting at the top of the neck, work your thumbs down and up the grooves. Drop and lift your elbows a little to allow your thumbs to come together.

4 Repeat the neck-warming technique to complete the routine.

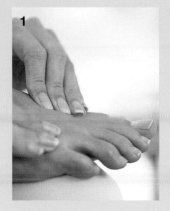

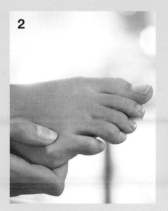

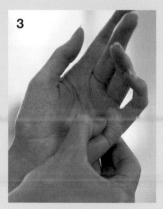

Tension release for shoulders

1 Stand behind the seated receiver with your feet turned out and legs supporting the back. With your fingers pointing down the back, ask them to breathe in. On the out breath, apply three palm presses using both hands simultaneously. Work from the neck to the edges of the shoulders.

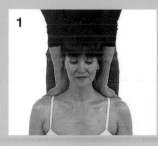

2 Reverse your hands so that your fingers are pointing down the chest. Return back to the neck, repeating the palm presses.

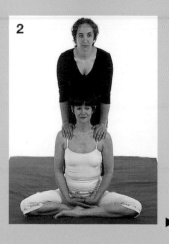

▶

Western massage

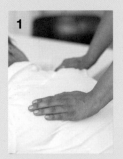

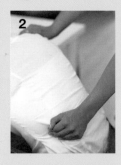

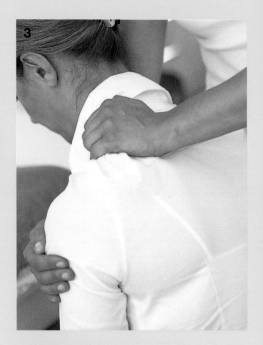

Neck and upper back routine

1 The receiver should be sitting at a table or desk, with the arms and upper body cushioned. Begin by resting your right hand on the receiver's right shoulder. Then, using your left hand, work from the left of the spine outwards, applying steady pressure from the heel of the hand and slowly moving from the lower back up to the top of the shoulder blade.

2 Make a fist with the working hand and work effleurage in large circles, applying the pressure on the upward strokes towards the heart.

3 Move side-on to the receiver, bring them more upright and move your right hand from the right shoulder across to the upper left arm, giving support across the front of the upper torso. With your left hand, lift and squeeze the muscle between the left shoulder blade and the spine with the heel of your hand and fingers. Move to the other side and repeat Steps 1–3.

4 Ask the receiver to drop their head slightly and, still supporting the front of the shoulders, squeeze the muscles of the neck between your fingers and thumb, working up towards the skull. 'Ground' the receiver by gently squeezing down the arms and legs to the feet.

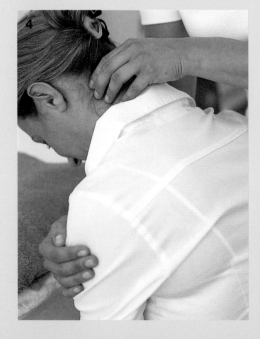

Shiatsu

Stiffness in the neck and shoulder area can be treated by working on the local area.

- Work on the *tsubos* in the neck and shoulder area in descending numerical order, starting with SI 15 and ending with SI 9 (see page 25).

- Facing the receiver, kneel astride the head and apply pressure to the area between SI 9 and SI 10 with your thumb. Repeat on the other shoulder.

- Use the palming technique to apply pressure between the shoulder blades with one hand or both hands simultaneously.

- Use the thumbing technique to work down the main inner course of the bladder meridian, which runs about 4 cm (1.5 in) away from the centre line of the back, up to the shoulder blades. Work in reverse in the same way, but this time along the outside branch of the meridian, which runs about 7.5 cm (3 in) from the centre line.

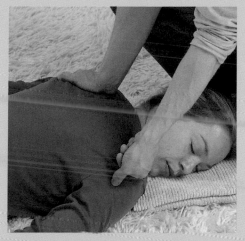

Working on the small intestine *tsubo*

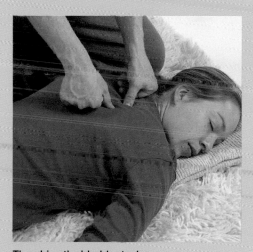

Thumbing the bladder *tsubo*

Frozen shoulder

If you have a pain in your shoulder as if you have slept awkwardly and then suddenly cannot lift your arm, and if every time you try to lift it you feel a deep burning pain and have no strength, you have a frozen shoulder. This is caused by injury or repetitive exercise, and those over the age of 40 are more susceptible. Specialists stress the importance of early help, and massage can offer effective treatments.

Quick fix

This simple technique will help ease the pain in the shoulder:

- Working on each shoulder in turn, use the fingers and thumb of one hand to press firmly around the shoulder blade, pressing in towards the blade. Use your other hand to support the shoulder.

Western massage
Soft tissue and tendon stretch

1 In a standing position, support the receiver's upper arm with both hands and place one hand on the underside of the shoulder joint, lifting it very slightly. Move gently to avoid pain.

2 Keeping one hand under the arm, slide your other hand down to the wrist for support and pull the straight arm forwards and outwards to a comfortable point of resistance.

3 Keeping your hands in the same position as in Step 2, pull outwards with the hand under the shoulder, at the same time pulling down with the hand supporting the wrist. Hold the stretch for as long as the receiver can bear, then release.

Thai massage
Relieving tension in the shoulders

1 The receiver should lie on one side with the lower leg extended straight and the upper leg bent in front of them at a right angle to the body. Kneel beside them, facing the head, close enough so that the back is supported against your thigh. Lift the upper arm and hook it over your inside arm. Clasp both your hands over the top of the shoulder.

2 Lean back with straight arms and gently pull the shoulder towards you, then rotate very slowly three times in each direction, using your body weight. The receiver should not hold their head off the floor as you pull, but let it hang and rise naturally with the stretch.

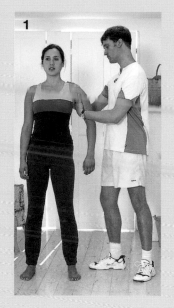

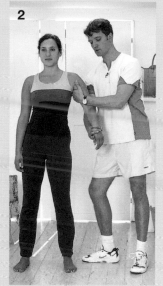

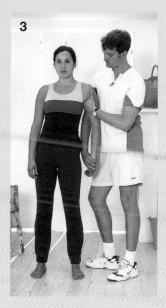

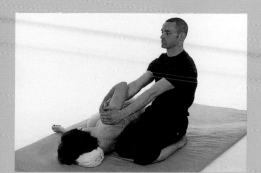

Rotating the shoulder

3 Bend your inside arm at the elbow to raise and support the receiver's arm at a right angle, allowing the trapezius muscles to relax. With the fingers of both hands, make circles along the trapezius line.

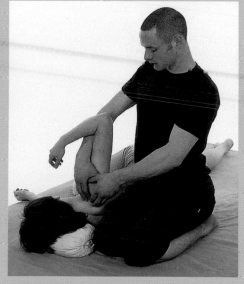

Massaging the trapezius

Reflexology

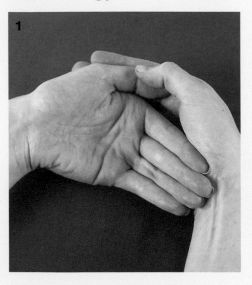

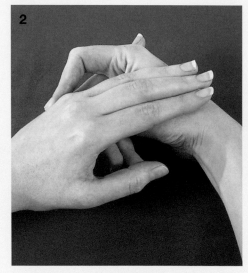

Five-reflex routine

1 To work on the neck reflex, cup one thumb in the other hand so that it is resting between your index and middle fingers, then use your working thumb to walk along the bone of the thumb from the first to the second joint (see page 20). Make seven small steps along the bone to represent the seven vertebrae in the neck.

2 To work on the shoulder reflex, place one hand palm downwards and place your working index finger and thumb between the base of the ring and little fingers. Apply pressure and, using the bird's beak technique, take three tiny steps towards the wrist, stimulating with small circles.

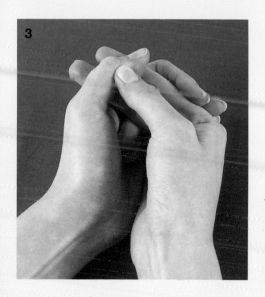

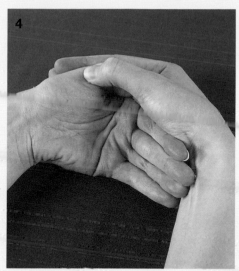

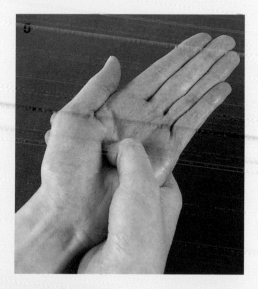

3 To work on the occipital bone reflex, place your working thumb against the first joint of the other thumb, hook up against the bone and stimulate in clockwise or anticlockwise circles.

4 To work on the upper spine reflex, cup one hand in the other, so that your working thumb rests on the bone at the base of the thumb. Make 12 small steps along the bone to the edge of the wrist, to represent the 12 vertebrae in the upper spine. Stimulate with small circles at each step.

5 To work on the kidney/adrenal glands reflex, support one hand in the other and place your working thumb in the webbing between the thumb and index finger, just above the thumb muscle halfway down the hand. Use your thumb to hook into the webbing and apply pressure.

Painful joints

Joints are formed where two or more bones meet. Movement is helped along by a lubricant called synovial fluid. Massage stimulates the production of this fluid, which is why sedentary and elderly people find regular treatments really help their mobility. One of the most common conditions found in the elderly is arthritis or joint disease. Inflammation of one or more joints is characterized by stiffness, pain and swelling, which again can be eased by massage.

Quick fix

In this reciprocal technique, benefiting both the giver and receiver, the giver has their back massaged while easing the receiver's hip, knee and ankle joints:

- The receiver should lie flat on the floor on their back, while you kneel close to their hips. Ask them to rest their feet on your ribcage, then walk them up and down the muscles on either side of your spine several times. Lean back into their feet, easing their knees open, and hold for two or three breaths. Release slightly and repeat three times.

Western massage

Hand and foot joint sequence

1 With the receiver's arm well supported, place your hand on the outside of the arm and, using petrissage, work up the forearm, squeezing the muscle between the heel of your hand and your fingers. Ease off the pressure over the joint area, then continue along the upper arm to the shoulder and return to the wrist.

2 Starting just above the wrist with your thumb on top of the forearm, glide the thumb pad up to the elbow, twist your hand around and return with the fingers gliding down the underneath of the arm. Repeat each movement three to five times.

3 Work over the back of the hand using the thumb pads to make slow, tiny circles, making sure that the hand and wrist are well supported. Repeat Steps 1–3 with the other arm.

4 With the leg well supported and one hand placed under and around the heel to take the weight of the foot, work over the whole of the top of the foot using the thumb pads to make slow, tiny circles.

5 Facing along the receiver's body, hold the ankle firmly with one hand, and with the other, push on the toes and ball of the foot until you reach a comfortable resistance point. Hold for five to ten seconds.

6 Place your hand on top of the foot and gradually pull downwards while pushing the heel with your other hand to a comfortable resistance point. Repeat Steps 5 and 6 five times each, then finish off with a gentle stroking movement from the ankle to the toes before working on the other foot.

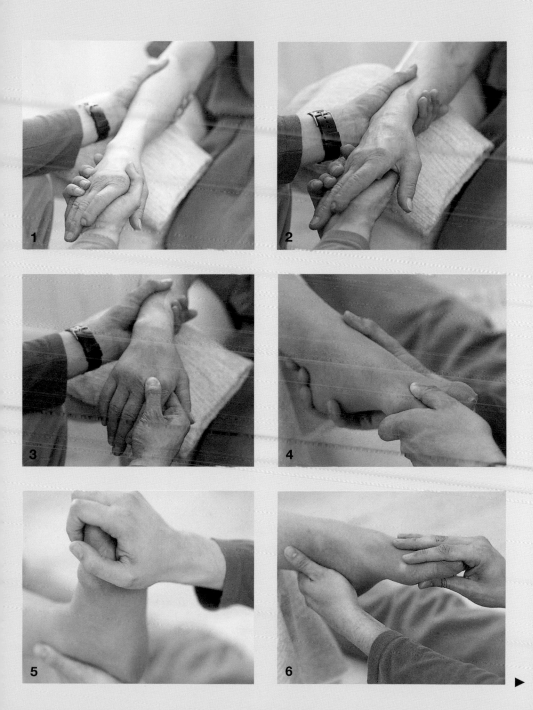

Reflexology

Hand reflexology is a very effective treatment for easing painful joints.

- To help relieve an arthritic hip, work on the whole musculoskeletal system, paying special attention to the hip joint point just above the wrist on the edge of the hand on the little finger side (see page 21).

- For stiff, painful knees, work on the knee point slightly further up the hand. Don't risk aggravating the pain by lingering on these points for too long – you just want to stimulate the energy flow.

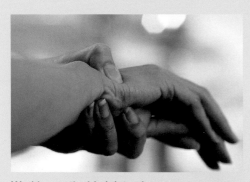

Working on the hip joint point

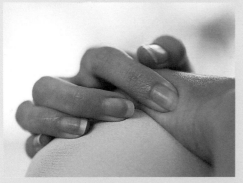

Working on the knee point

Thai massage

Easing stiffness in the fingers and wrist

1 Hold the receiver's wrist gently with one hand and lace your fingers through theirs with the other. Rotate the wrist three times in each direction, then slide your fingers out.

2 Still supporting the wrist, take each finger in turn and hold it between your second and third fingers as shown. Rotate each finger in turn in both directions loosely, and finally grip and at the same time slowly slide stretch the finger. It may 'pop' as you stretch it, but this is nothing to be concerned about.

Shiatsu

Relieving stiff joints

1 In a kneeling position at the side of the receiver's leg, lay the leg over your thigh to support it. Work down the inner thigh using the palming technique, with your fingers turned towards you, following the spleen meridian down to the ankle (see page 24).

2 Use the thumbing technique to work on the *tsubos* along the spleen meridian, again working down the leg from the inner thigh. The important ones are Sp 10, the width of two thumbs above the knee starting from the inner edge of the kneecap, Sp 9, on the inside of the calf, just under the bulge of bone below the side of the knee, Sp 6, four finger-widths up the inner leg from the ankle bone, starting from the fleshy area behind the ankle bone, and Sp 3, on the side of the foot just behind the main joint of the big toe.

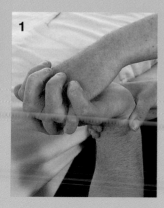

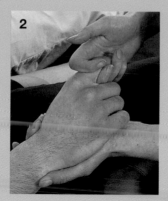

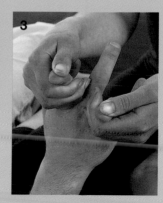

3 Starting in the centre of the palm, knead and push the fingers back using your thumbs in the caterpillar style. Start with the thumb and little finger simultaneously and walk inwards to the next two fingers, as shown, followed by the centre finger.

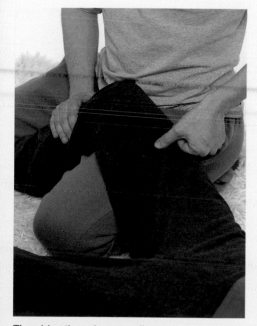

Thumbing the spleen merdian

Acupressure

For knee pain, spread the hand with the middle finger on the middle of the outer edge of the kneecap, working on St 34 above the knee, and St 36 outside the knee and Sp 9 and 10 on the inner side (see page 24). Rubbing this area also stimulates the right points – St 34, 35 and 36. Massage around the outside of the joint. Do the same around all painful joints.

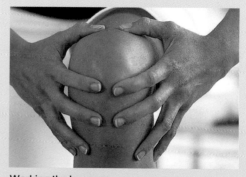

Working the kneecap

Tired feet

We spend a surprising amount of our everyday lives standing on our feet, yet we often take their wellbeing for granted. If you have a job that involves a great deal of standing or walking, there is nothing as revitalizing as a foot massage – it's also a great way to end a hard day's shopping!

Quick fixes

Try these simple techniques to aid rapid relaxation of the feet:

- Hold the foot so that one hand is on the sole and one on top. Working from the ankles to the toes, massage it with long, firm strokes.

- Holding the heel in one hand and the toes in the other, circle five times clockwise, then anticlockwise.

- Starting at the heel, use your thumb to press along the inside edge of the foot all the way up to the big toe. Press firmly and follow the line up over the instep. Then repeat on the outside edge of the foot, from the heel to the little toe.

Western massage

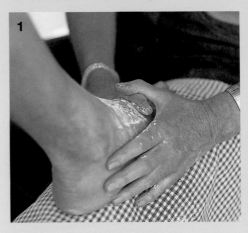

Foot revitalizing routine

1 Apply talcum powder to aid the glide and light pressure of this massage. Place the flat of your hands on the top of the foot, with one thumb on top of the other, ready to do the effleurage stroke. On your out breath, work up the front of the foot towards the lower leg. When you reach this point, glide back down on either side of the foot, leaning back to add a slight pull to the stroke. Repeat three or four times.

Thai massage
Foot soothing routine

1 Working both feet at the same time, and starting at Point 1 on the diagram, thumb press along the points shown towards the ball of the foot and back again. Rock your body weight on and off the thumb very slowly.

2 Finish the sequence with an alternate palm press of the feet.

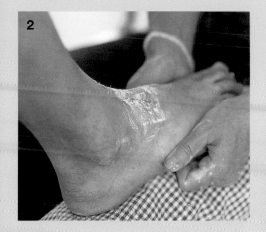

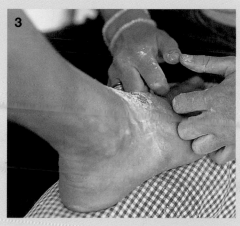

2 From a position that enables you to keep your arms straight, rest your thumbs and the heel of your hands on the top of the foot, with your fingers wrapped around the sides. Draw your thumbs across the foot in opposite directions, squeezing the foot firmly, and bring them down to join the rest of your hand in a movement that stretches and opens up the area.

3 Apply the knuckling stroke, circling all over the top and sides of the foot. Repeat several times. Now use the same strokes on the other foot. At the end of the routine, hold the receiver's foot for 20 seconds to 'ground' them.

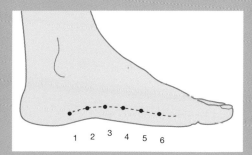

Medial arch points

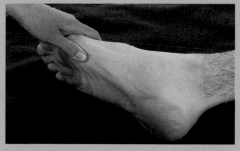

Applying thumb presses to the medial arch

Repetitive strain injury

Repetitive strain injury (RSI) is a health problem relating to the workplace. It is a collective term used for carpel tunnel syndrome, non-specific arm pain, occupational overuse and disorders of the upper arm. Although often associated with using a computer keyboard, it can be caused by any repetitive action. It can affect the hands, arms, neck and shoulders, and symptoms include pain, stiffness, pins and needles, swelling, numbness and loss of manual dexterity.

Quick fixes

Use these techniques with your partner to give one another speedy, after-work relief:

- Place your thumbs together on one of the receiver's forearms and slowly and steadily spread them outwards, applying a gentle pressure. Repeat over the rest of the forearm, then switch to the other arm.

- Use the effleurage stroke down the back of the neck and over the shoulder area.

- Press firmly with your thumbs over the hands, then draw your fingers between the receiver's fingers.

Reflexology

To release the twinges and soreness of repetitive strain injury in your hands, arms or shoulders, try the following foot techniques. (See pages 92–93 for a hand reflexology routine that can also be used for RSI.)

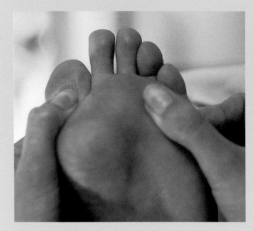

Working on the shoulder girdle

Acupressure
Treatment for RSI

1 Run an index finger up and down the sides of the fingers, pull each finger and thumb, then lightly press your nail around all the fingernails and the thumbnail.

2 With the palm facing upwards, tap firmly 12 times up the forearm, then tap the inside of the elbow 12 times. Turn the arm over and tap the other side of the elbow too.

- Start by working on the musculoskeletal and nervous systems on the feet (see pages 19 and 20). Then concentrate on the neck, under the big toe, and the shoulder girdle, below the little toe. Then work on the arm reflex, running down the edge of the foot from the little toe to the midpoint, and the hand reflex, just off-centre on the sole on the little toe side, just below the ball. Move on to the hip and leg reflexes, down the lower half of the edge of the foot on the little toe side.

- To break the stress-holding patterns, do extra work on the finger and toe joints, rotating and stretching them gently.

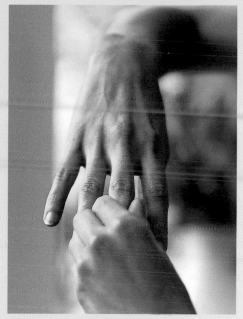

Rotating and stretching the finger joints

3 Gently massage across the fold at the inside of the elbow, from the point on the heart meridian at the spot where the fold ends when your arm is bent, across the centre (see page 24). These are points for releasing the energy stagnation that occurs with RSI.

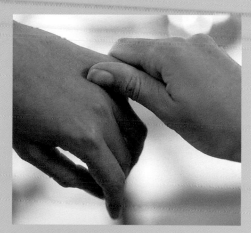

Pulling the fingers ▶

Western massage

Hands and wrist treatment

1 Using the pads of your thumbs and rotating them alternately in opposite directions, work in between and over the bony area of the wrist.

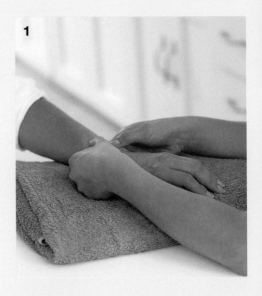

2 Starting with the heel of your hands on the centre back of the receiver's hand, apply pressure and glide them in opposite directions across to the edge, where your fingers are wrapped around the receiver's hand. This will really stretch and open up the area. Repeat this step three to five times.

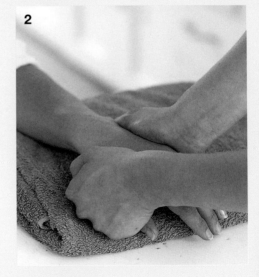

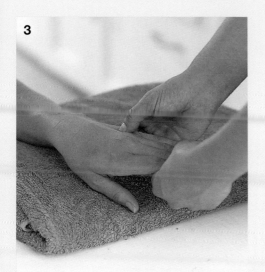

3 Holding the receiver's hand, place your thumb pad just above the web between the third and fourth fingers, then apply pressure and glide up towards the wrist, following the hollow channel between the knuckles. Move to the web between the second and third fingers and repeat the movement, continuing in this way until you have worked all four areas on the receiver's hand.

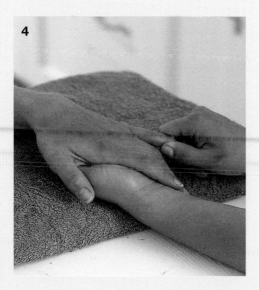

4 Supporting the receiver's hand in a flat, handshake-type clasp, take the little finger at the base between your thumb and index finger and gently slide down, stretching and twisting as you go and pulling off at the tip. Move along the hand, working each finger and the thumb. Move to the other hand and repeat Steps 1–4.

Maximizing the benefit

Use a little massage oil to help maintain smooth, flowing movements. Alternatively, use a favourite hand cream, which will have the added benefit of rehydrating the skin at the same time.

Tennis elbow

This is caused by tightness and overstraining of the wrist extensors or by nodules and lesions that make the muscles prone to injury. The initial sign is an ache in the mid-section of the forearm, which recurs each time there is activity of the arm and wrist. In the worst case, the wrist, not the elbow, needs to be immobilized for a period of time, but usually massage and manipulation of the joints will relieve the complaint.

Quick fix

Try this simple reflexology technique to relieve the problem:

- Locate the elbow point on the foot, which is on the small bony protrusion halfway down the outer edge of the foot (see page 20). Press on this with your index finger for five seconds, then gradually release.

Western massage
Three-step therapy

1 Facing the receiver, support the arm with your forearm and hold the elbow in your hand.

2 Place your thumb on the outside of the elbow with your fingers underneath to apply counter pressure and, working around the outside of the elbow, apply pressure with the pad of your thumb, rotating it at the same time.

3 Now use the tip of your thumb instead of the pad to apply pressure by moving it back and forth across the elbow in short strokes. Continue for one to two minutes, or to the receiver's tolerance level, as this can cause discomfort.

Shiatsu
Treatment for tennis elbow

1 The receiver should lie on their side, with their arm gently resting against their body. Place one hand on their shoulder as support, then use the heel of your hand to work down the large intestine meridian from the upper arm and along the edge of the forearm to the wrist (see page 25).

2 Work down the meridian using your thumb, again from the upper arm, past the elbow and along the forearm to the wrist, paying particular attention to point LI 11. This is located at the end of the fold at the elbow on top of the elbow joint.

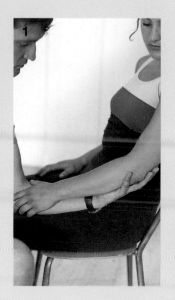
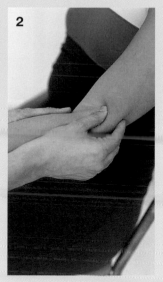
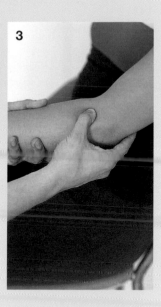

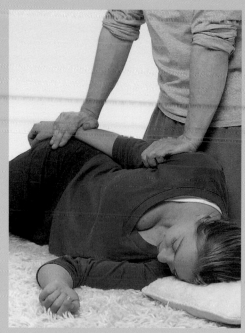

Palming the large intestine merdian

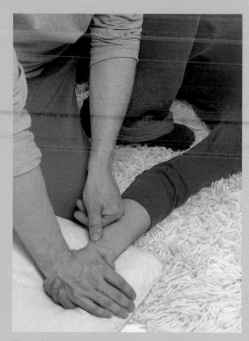

Thumbing the large intestine meridian ▶

Reflexology

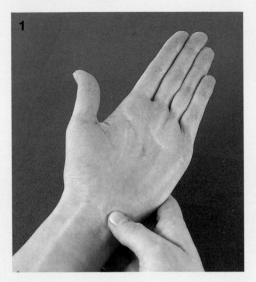

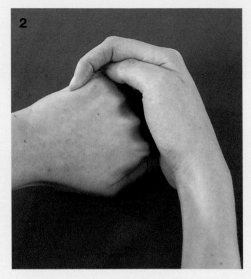

Tennis elbow/RSI routine

1 Place your working thumb at one side of the wrist and thumb-walk at the base of the hand from one side of the wrist to the other. Stimulate with small circles at each step. Repeat.

2 Place one hand palm downwards, then place your working index finger at the side of the hand just at the base of the little finger. Make two tiny steps towards the wrist with your index finger and tear back towards the fingers.

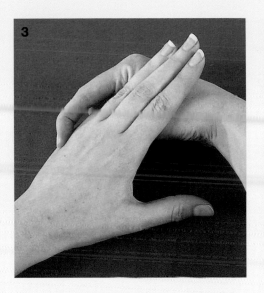

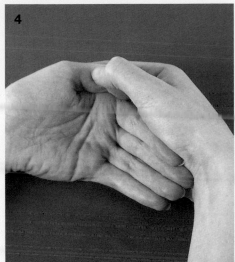

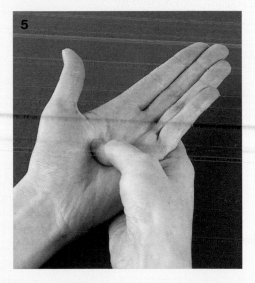

3 Place one hand palm downwards, then place your working index finger and thumb between the bases of the ring and little fingers. Apply pressure and use the bird's beak technique to take three tiny steps towards the wrist and stimulate with small circles.

4 Cup one thumb in the other hand so that it is resting between your index and middle fingers, then use your working thumb to walk along the bone of the thumb from the first to the second joint. Make seven small steps along the bone, to represent the seven vertebrae in the neck.

5 Support one hand in the other, then place your working thumb in the webbing between the thumb and index finger just above the thumb muscle halfway down the hand. Use your thumb to hook into the webbing and apply pressure.

Muscle cramps

Calf cramps are muscle contractions that send the calf into spasm, and they may occur for no obvious reason. They can be alleviated with a simple kneading stroke, which can also be adapted for self-massage (see Western massage routine, right).

Quick fixes

Use these techniques for the rapid relief of muscular cramp in the calves:

- To ease the pain, press with your index finger or thumb on point GB 34, which is just below the knee (see page 25). Feel for a dip between the large shin bone, the tibia and the smaller fibula. It is just below the knobbly top of the tibia.

- To ease the contraction, gently knead the muscles of the calves.

Western massage

Kneading and stretching routine

1 With fingers together, cup both hands around the back of the calf so that the tips of the fingers are facing each other along the midline of the calf muscle. Exert pressure with both hands simultaneously and roll the muscle using the kneading stroke, then release the pressure and repeat, slowly moving your hands up the calf to reduce the muscle tension and relieve spasm.

2 Supporting the ankle, flex the foot to its point of resistance by pushing the toes and ball of the foot forward with the other hand. Then pull back the foot with one hand, while pushing down on the heel with the other. This will stretch the calf muscle and increase blood flow to the area.

Thai massage

Try these techniques to release tension in the calf muscles. The receiver may laugh as a release of ticklishness.

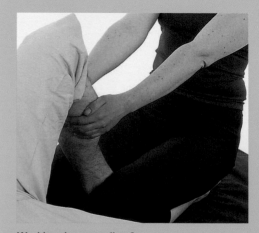

Working down *sen* line 2

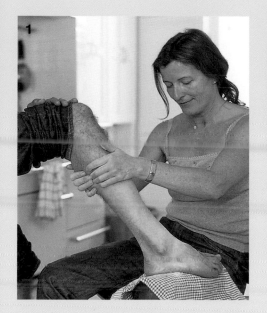

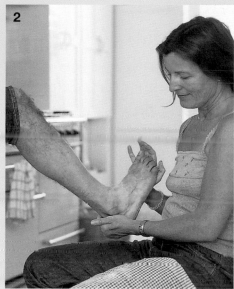

- Hook your fingertips into the central *sen* line (*sen* line 2, see page 30) on the back of the calf at the knee. Lean back and slowly pull inwards, then outwards, with both hands simultaneously, three or four times, travelling down the line.

- Walk back up the line using alternate hands.

- Interlacing your fingers, clasp the receiver's calf muscle with your palms. Press the sides of the calf muscle firmly with the heels of your hands and push the muscle away from you. Work from the knee down to the lower calf and back up.

- Finish by shaking the calf gently with the thumb and index finger.

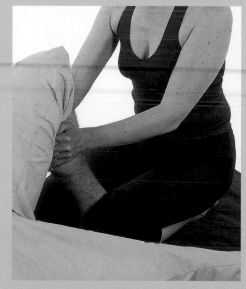

Interlacing the calf muscle

Poor circulation

Many people suffer from poor circulation, especially when they grow older. This results in cold and numbness in the hands and feet as well as stiffness. Massage improves the flow of blood to these areas. It also helps the circulation by aiding the effective drainage of muscle tissues.

Quick fix

Try this quick acupressure technique to improve the circulation of blood around the body:

- Work on point Bl 23 on the bladder meridian by placing your hands on the waist with your thumbs on the big muscles beside the spine (see page 25).

Western massage

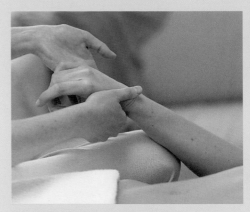

Warming and draining the hands

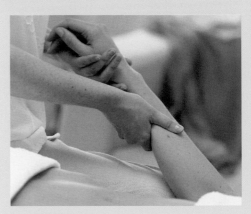

Draining the arms

Work on these areas of the body regularly to improve circulation and muscle drainage.

- To combat cold and numbness in the hands, rub the hands together vigorously, then shake them. Grasp each finger in turn and squeeze down its length to warm it up. Then lift each finger upwards and backwards to drain back down the hand towards the wrist.

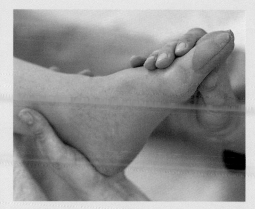

Boosting circulation to the feet

- With the arm well supported, use your fingers and thumbs to apply pressure down the forearm to the elbow, to help facilitate drainage. Repeat with the other arm.

- Place your hand on the top of the foot with your thumb underneath. Use your thumb to make slow, tiny circles across the sole, starting at the heel and ending at the ball of the foot. Use firm, even pressure so that you don't tickle the receiver. Support the heel and ankle with the other hand. Repeat with the other foot.

- To treat swollen ankles, aid drainage by applying pressure upwards around each ankle in the direction of the calf.

Shiatsu

Heart meridian massage

1 The receiver should lie on their back, arms loosely by their sides, with the palms facing upwards. Half-kneel over one arm and grasp it at the top, by the armpit. Using the palming technique, work down the heart meridian to the elbow, then continue down the forearm to the wrist, projecting more weight onto the thumb side (see page 24).

2 With the receiver lying on their side, use the thumbing technique to work along the meridian again, continuing down the palm to the little finger. Apply gentle pressure to both sides of the finger, working down to the tip.

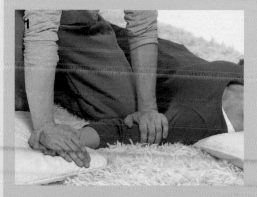

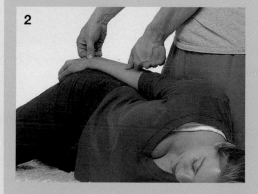

Digestive problems

Indigestion is the incomplete digestion of foods in the stomach. Symptoms include heartburn, nausea, bloating, passing wind, abdominal pain and a sensation of fullness. Stress can inhibit the abdominal blood supply, leading to indigestion and an adverse effect on the absorption and distribution of nutrients. In addition, the muscle wall of the intestinal tract, which pushes the food through the body by contracting, cannot function properly. Massage can be highly useful in tackling these problems.

Quick fix

Use this simple technique to ease tension in the stomach:

- Position the fingers of one hand so that they are pointing towards the area just below your ribcage. Gradually lean forwards to apply increasing pressure to the area. Be sure to exhale as you lean forwards, then inhale as you draw back. Repeat several times.

Western massage

Soothing and stretching the abdomen

1 Use the effleurage stroke to glide from the abdomen to just under the breast area and then, with your hands on either side of the torso, slowly return to your starting position. Repeat five times in a flowing movement. This will calm and soothe abdominal bloating and indigestion.

2 After you have relaxed the area in Step 1, using the flat of your hands and gentle pressure, on the receiver's out breath, draw your hands apart diagonally (left ribs to right hip, for example), working outwards in a sweeping, stretching action. Repeat in the other direction.

Reflexology

For digestive problems in general, work with the whole digestive tract, starting from the mouth and following right through to the rectum.

- Points to concentrate on include the liver and gall bladder, located in the right hand (see page 20).

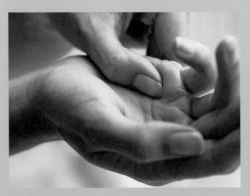

Working on the liver reflex

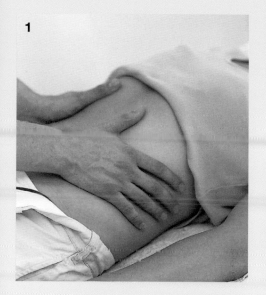

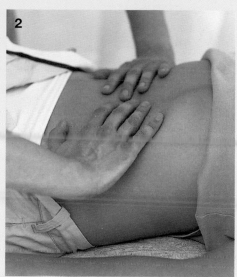

- If you have cramping stomach pains, work on the thyroid and parathyroid reflexes between the thumb and index finger on the front of the hands, plus the diaphragm and the solar plexus in the palms.

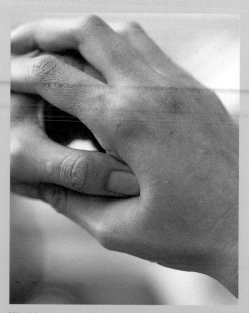

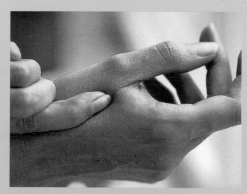

Working on the thyroid reflex

Working on the parathyroid reflex

Reflexology

Hand routine for digestive disorders

1 Support one hand in the other and place your working thumb at the tip of the webbing. Then walk to the edge of the hand and return back to your original point. Continue in this manner until you have covered the entire area of the webbing, rather like the spokes of a bicycle wheel.

2 Place your working thumb a third of the way down the palm of your other hand. Use the butterfly movement to walk across the hand from one side to the other.

3 Place your working thumb on the diaphragm line between zones 2 and 3 (see page 17) and apply a firm pressure.

4 Place your working thumb on the hiatus hernia point, as shown, and walk up between the bones to the bases of the index and middle fingers. Continue in this manner, stimulating with small circles at each step.

5 Place your working thumb on the diaphragm line at the joint at the base of the middle finger. Use your thumb to hook up towards the ring finger and against the joint.

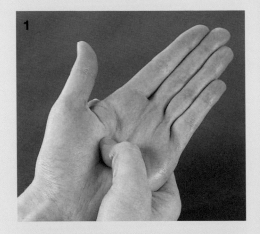

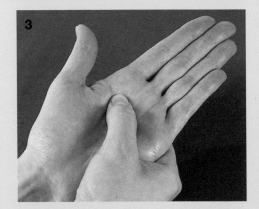

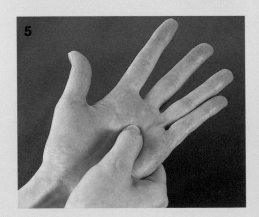

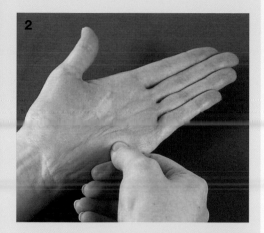

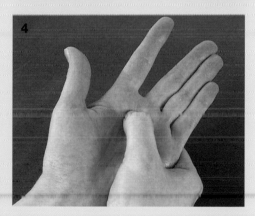

Acupressure

Try these strategies for treating any minor digestive problems.

- For heartburn, work on point CV 12, on the conception vessel, and LI 4, between the finger and thumb (see pages 24–25). Press your thumb against the first finger and see where the webbing bulges up highest then put your other thumb on that point, letting the first thumb open out away from the hand, and hold that point with finger and thumb.

- Indigestion is eased by working on St 36. Find a bump just below your kneecap, towards the outside leg, measure three finger-widths down the bone and press.

- Stomach massage also helps. Early in the morning is the best time to massage the abdomen, because the stomach meridian is most active between 7 and 9am.

Stressed stomach

The abdomen is the most exposed and unprotected area of the body, and it is also the place in which we store our deepest emotions. When massaging this area, be aware that the receiver may feel vulnerable, so take time to observe their breathing pattern and try to coordinate your strokes with this.

Quick fix

Try this easy head massage technique to soothe a stressed stomach:

- Place the end pad of one finger on the tip of the nose. Within the bounds of reasonable comfort, press as hard as you can and rotate slowly for 30 seconds.

Reflexology

Digestive system routine

1 Support one hand in the other and place your working thumb at the tip of the webbing. Then walk to the edge of the hand and return back to your original point. Continue in this manner until you have covered the entire area of the webbing, rather like the spokes of a bicycle wheel.

2 To work on the liver (right hand) or spleen (left hand) reflex, place your working thumb on the edge of the hand, one thumbprint down from the base of the little finger. Using the thumb-walking technique, take three small steps into the hand. Continue in this manner for four lines, finishing just above the wrist.

3 Place your working thumb at the base of zone 4 just above the wrist (see page 17). Turn your thumbnail so that it faces up to the ring finger. Walk up zone 4 until halfway up the hand. Push down and stimulate before turning to walk across the hand, finishing between the webbing.

Thai massage

Relaxing a stressed stomach

1 Kneel down with your knees wide apart, with your body weight resting on your knees, your buttocks raised and your toes flexed. Position yourself as close as possible to the receiver.

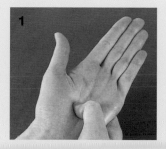

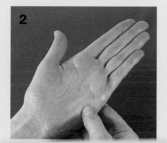

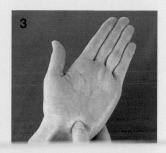

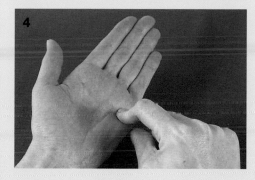

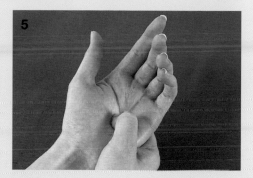

4 Place your working index finger and thumb two finger-widths from the base of the fingers. Apply pressure and walk with tiny steps across the hand. Continue in this manner over the palm until you reach the wrist.

5 Place your working thumb in the centre of the palm and relax your hand so that the fingers fall over the working thumb. Apply pressure and stimulate with small circles, taking deep breaths.

2 With one hand placed over the other, very gently circle the *hara*, the area that lies between the ribs and diaphragm down to the hip bones and the pubic bone, with the navel as the centre. Move in a clockwise direction. The upper hand is used as the mother hand only (see page 27).

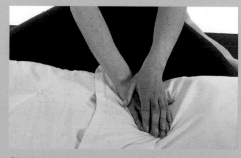

Circling the *hara*

Nausea/travel sickness

Feeling sick and vomiting can have a wide variety of causes, including stomach bugs, food intolerance, motion and drug side-effects.
If you have eaten something that has caused the sickness, vomiting is the natural, healthy response as the body tries to get rid of it, so this should not be prevented. But massage can help to relieve the unpleasant sensation of nausea and to rebalance the digestive tract after a bout of vomiting.

Quick fix

Work this acupressure point if you start to feel nauseous:

- Stimulate point Liv 13 at the side and bottom of the ribcage, in line with the hip bone (see page 24).

Western massage

The following two techniques help to relax the whole abdominal area and are also comforting.

- Work on the receiver's back, making large circular movements in an anticlockwise direction with your hands flat and applying a medium pressure. Keep the movements smooth and soothing.

- Using one hand, make a series of small circular movements with your fingers over the abdomen in a large circle, moving in a clockwise direction. Keep the movements smooth and slow, to induce relaxation, and the pressure light.

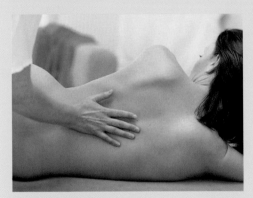

Circling the back

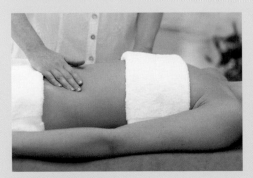

Circling the abdomen

Reflexology

There are various reflexology techniques to treat different aspects of sickness:

- To restore the digestive system after vomiting, finger-walk down the oesophagus reflex on the foot, gently press and rotate on the stomach area and work both ways over the intestines (see page 18). Finish by working the colon and rectum. Use plenty of soothing massage strokes between working on the specific areas.

- To treat travel sickness, start by working on the whole digestive system as above, but use hand reflexology if you are self-massaging so that you don't cramp your stomach while working on your foot (see page 20). Return to the solar plexus and pituitary gland points, rotating your thumb on them. Thumb-walk across the diaphragm and the middle and upper spine.

- To treat the stomach area in particular, finger-walk down the centre of the right foot. Again, you can use this technique on your left hand instead if self-massaging.

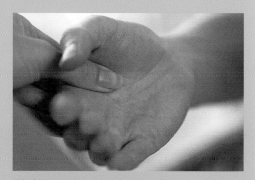

Working on the solar plexus reflex

Acupressure

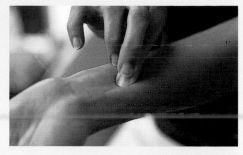

Working on point Pc 6

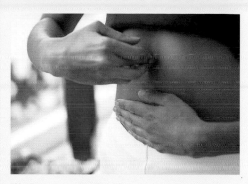

Working on point CV 12

Acupressure offers some simple, effective remedies for both sickness and nausea:

- Pc 6 is the most reliable energy remedy for all kinds of sickness, so much so that it is even used in hospitals (see page 24). Three finger-widths up from the wrist, press with the third finger, right in the centre of the inner arm (for many people, this is under the buckle of their watch strap). You can buy wrist straps that work this point for travel sickness.

- A point that is very effective in easing the feelings of nausea is CV 12, in the centre of the abdomen.

Constipation

If you suffer from constipation, you will be well aware of its effects on your body. It is one of the main causes of sluggishness and lack of energy. It also leads to a build-up of large amounts of toxins, which results in lacklustre skin and eyes and unpleasant-smelling breath.

Quick fix

Try this easy head massage technique:

- Find the indent in your chin, then rotate as firmly as you can bear for 30 seconds. Vigorous massaging of this area will greatly help rectify the condition and also bring back life and colour to your complexion.

Acupressure

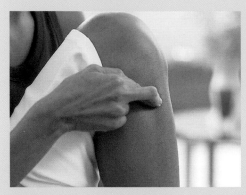

Working on the 'three-mile' point

Constipation can be greatly eased by the following acupressure treatments.

- Work on point St 36: find a bump just below your kneecap, towards the outside leg, then measure three finger-widths down the bone and press (see page 24). This is known as the 'three-mile' point.

- Working on point LI 4, also known as the 'great eliminator', is excellent for treating constipation. Press your thumb against the first finger and see where the webbing bulges up highest. Put your other thumb on that point, then – letting the first thumb open out away from the hand – hold that point with finger and thumb.

Reflexology

Target these areas to help treat constipation:

- Work on the colon, which is most easily done on the hands – it runs across the palm from the thumb side a couple of finger-widths up from the wrist (see page 20).

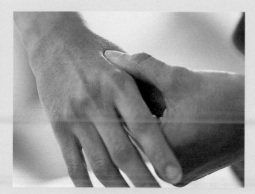

Working on the 'great eliminator'

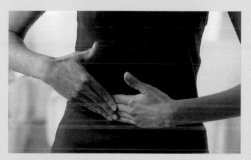

Massaging the stomach

- Stomach massage will also help – work in a clockwise direction from CV 6 in small circular movements. It is worth massaging the stomach before you go to bed so that the effects take place overnight.

- Work on the area along the back of the ankle and the heel on the Achilles tendon, known as the 'chronic helper'.

Western massage

You will find this movement especially helpful in relieving constipation. Remember to follow the receiver's breath with your hands.

- With the receiver lying flat on their back, place one hand on top of the other and, making sure that your whole hand is in contact with the receiver, work in a circular, clockwise movement from the solar plexus, following the direction of the large intestine (see diagram below). Start with a large circle and continue, reducing the size of the circle but increasing the pressure, for a further four or five times.

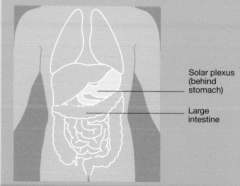

Solar plexus
(behind
stomach)

Large
intestine

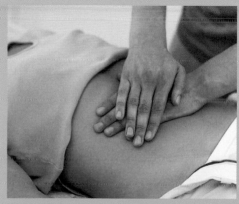

Circling from the solar plexus

PMT and menstrual pain

By inducing relaxation, massage can reduce the symptoms of premenstrual tension, such as tension, irritability, depression and crying spells. It can also release tightness in muscles and stimulate the blood and lymph flows, thereby helping in the elimination of toxins and excess fluid. It is, however, very important to work within the comfort level of the receiver, as sometimes the body may feel too tense and sensitive for anything other than very light strokes.

Quick fixes

Try these speedy techniques to bring you quick relief from PMT and menstrual pain:

- Measure up from the top of one ankle about three finger-widths. Apply firm pressure with your thumb over the bone.

- Rub your breasts to promote the upward flow of energy and stimulate the hormone prolactin, which helps ease menstrual pain.

Thai massage

Easing menstrual pain

1 Kneel down with your knees wide apart, with your body weight resting on the knees, your buttocks raised and your toes flexed. Position yourself as close as possible to the receiver. With one hand placed over the other, very gently circle the *hara*, which lies between the ribs and the diaphragm down to the hip bones and pubic bone, in a clockwise direction.

2 On the receiver's out breath, gently but firmly push the heels of both hands in the direction of the navel.

Western massage

This simple massage technique will help ease period pain:

- Make wide circles in an anticlockwise direction over the sacrum, the triangular bone at the base of the spine, and the lower back using the flat of your hand and following the contours of the body. This will have a warming, relaxing effect.

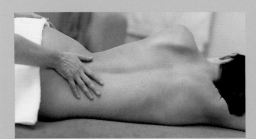

Circling the sacrum

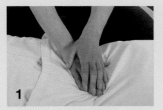

1 Circling the *hara*

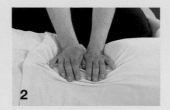

2 Pushing movement

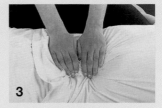

3 Pulling movement

3 Angle your hands so that the fingers are pointing downwards, then pull them towards the navel. Cup your hands over the navel and bring them back to the 'push' position above.

4 Repeat these push and pull movements several times until the *hara* area feels soft and relaxed. You may travel lower towards the hips and then higher towards the ribs.

5 Finish by making gentle circles over the *hara*, as at the start.

Caution
Do not use this routine on anyone who has had surgery in the last three months.

Acupressure

Use the following techniques to help you cope with heavy or painful periods.

- Work on points on the lower back, such as Bl 20–29. Put your hands on your waist, pressing your thumbs into the long muscles beside your spine, starting at waist level and working your way down to your hips. For extra effect, rotate your hips as you are pressing.

- Put the backs of your hands on your lower back to connect the bladder meridian with LI 4, the point between the finger and thumb, calming and opening the blood circulation in that area.

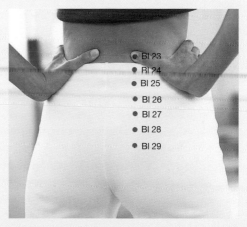

Working on points on the lower back

- Rubbing Sp 12 (in the crease where the front of the thigh joins the body, just beside the vulva), Sp 13 (close to Sp 12 but slightly farther towards the outside of the body) and CV 6 (below the navel) can help regulate periods and ease cramps.

▶

Reflexology

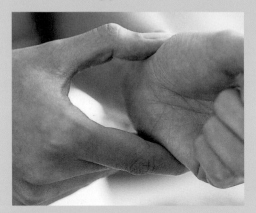

Working on the uterus

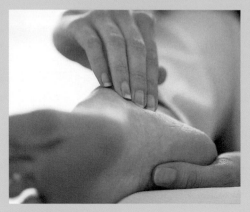

Working on the ovaries

Self-help is invaluable when you have PMT or heavy and painful periods. Working on your hands is soothing and accessible at any time of day, but working on the feet is just as effective.

- On the hands, work on the uterus, below the thumb just above the bump of bone, the ovaries, below the little fingers, and also the fallopian tubes, across the back of the wrist (see page 21).

- On the feet, work on the ovaries, on the outside of the heel, the pituitary, on the pad of the big toe, and the spine, including the lower back area, which runs down the edge of the foot from the big toe (see pages 18–20).

- Also work on the kidneys and ureter, on the soles of the feet, to remove any stress from other organs in that area.

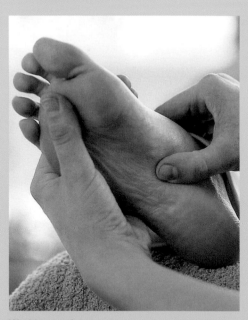

Working on the ureter

Reproductive system routine

1 Support one thumb on the fingers of your other hand. Use your working thumb to stimulate the centre of your other thumb.

2 Support one hand on the other and place your working thumb in the webbing between the thumb and index finger just above the thumb muscle halfway down the hand. Use your thumb to hook into the webbing and apply pressure to the point.

3 Place your working thumb at the base of the hand just above the wrist and walk along the bone towards the base of the thumb. Make five small steps to the edge of the hand, to represent the five vertebrae in the lumbar spine. Stimulate with small circles at each step.

4 To work the uterus/prostate reflex, place your hand palm downwards and use your working thumb to follow down the side of the hand from the thumb to the base of the wrist, where you will find a small indentation. Using the rotation-on-a-point technique, apply pressure to the point with your thumb.

5 To work on the ovaries/testes reflex, place your hand palm downwards and use your working index finger to follow down from the little finger to the base of the wrist, where you will find a small indentation. Using the rotation on-a-point technique, and rotating clockwise and then anticlockwise continually, apply pressure to the point with your index finger.

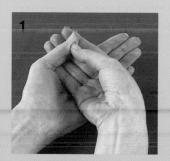
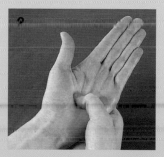
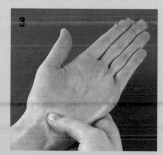
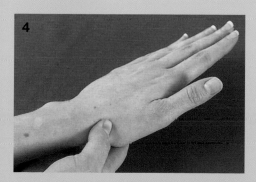
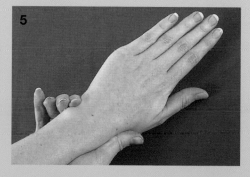

Early pregnancy

Although body massage must be avoided during the first 12 weeks of pregnancy, a head or face massage can be used to soothe away anxiety or headaches. Once this period has passed, massage techniques can be effective in combating the problem of morning sickness.

Quick fix

Try this simple technique:

- Stimulating the wrist is a reliable remedy for morning sickness – press with the third finger three finger-widths down the wrist in the centre of the forearm.

Caution

- Avoid body massage during the first 12 weeks.
- Avoid using deep pressure or vigorous strokes, especially on the abdomen, inner thigh and groin.
- Avoid applying pressure around and across the top of the ankles.
- Up to the 36th week, do not use essential oils in any form. Some oils are not suitable for use at any stage of pregnancy, so use a specially designed pre-mixed blend.

Shiatsu

Use this shiatsu technique to alleviate the problem of mornng sickness.

- The receiver should sit cross-legged, supported by a cushion. Kneel down, with knees wide apart, close to their back. Work down the bladder meridian, which runs down the back a couple of finger-widths away from the spine, by applying pressure with the thumb and the middle joint of the index finger (see page 25).

- Give particular attention to the central region, near the points for the liver, gall bladder, spleen and stomach (BI 18, BI 19 and BI 20).

Reflexology

These simple remedies for morning sickness are ideal for partners to learn, so that they can help women through pregnancy.

- Start by working the whole digestive system (see pages 18–20), concentrating on the oesophagus to ease nausea.

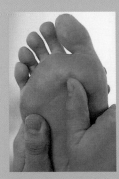

Working on the oesophagus

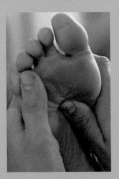

Working on the solar plexus

- Work on the pericardium meridian, particularly Pc 6, then the stomach meridian at points St 36 and 44, before applying steady pressure to Liv 3 (see page 24).

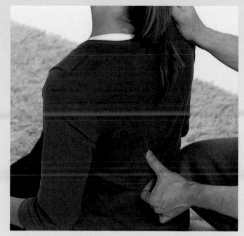

Caution
- Throughout pregnancy, do not apply strong pressure to the top of the receiver's shoulders.
- Do not work on points LI 4 and Sp 6 or the liver, spleen and kidney meridians below the knee.

Massaging the bladder meridian

- Return to the solar plexus and pituitary gland points, rotating your thumb on them. Thumb walk along the diaphragm and the middle and upper spine, and work some strips over the stomach area, which is mainly on the left foot.

- Include the endocrine system to help balance hormones.

Caution
Do not use reflexology in the first 16 weeks of pregnancy in case the changed flow of energy triggers a miscarriage, especially in a first pregnancy or if the woman has miscarried before.

Acupressure
This is a useful technique for early pregnancy:
- Rubbing up and down the conception vessel, down the centre of the body below the navel (see page 24), helps maintain a pregnancy if there was difficulty conceiving.

Caution
Do not use Sp 6 in pregnancy, and do not overwork the uterus and pituitary gland until the end of pregnancy.

Mid-pregnancy

Massage during the mid-stage of pregnancy becomes increasingly useful for easing lower backache as the weight of the baby begins to take its toll on the mother, as well as soothing other aches and pains. It is also excellent for reducing water retention and addressing any circulatory problems, particularly the common 'heavy leg' feelings.

Quick fix

This simple technique will give welcome comfort and reassurance:

- To relieve tension and strain, use a gentle effleurage stroke over the whole back.

Western massage

Leg and ankle sequence

1 Making sure that the receiver's back and legs are well supported, place the pads of both thumbs at the top of the shin on the outer edge of one leg, where the bone widens towards the knee, and apply comfortable pressure three to five times.

2 Moving down the leg, support the receiver's foot with one hand and place the thumb pad of the other hand about four finger-widths above the inner ankle bone, applying comfortable pressure three to five times. This movement induces calm and relaxation.

3 With one hand supporting the foot, take the small toe between your index finger and thumb and pull and squeeze in a downward movement, rotating the toe very slightly from the base to the tip. Apply to each toe. Repeat Steps 1–3 with the other leg. Finish by holding the feet for 30 seconds to 'ground' the receiver.

Reflexology

Reflexology is a boon for easing aches and pains as the pregnancy advances.

- Work on the entire reproductive as well as the musculoskeletal system (see pages 18–20) to bring effective relief to aching legs and back.

- A gentle all-over foot massage is a very soothing experience during the mid- to late stages of pregnancy.

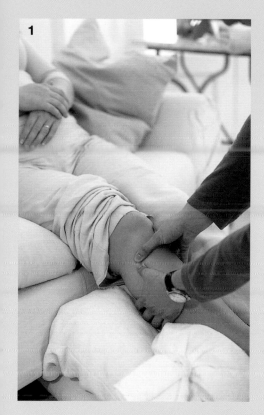

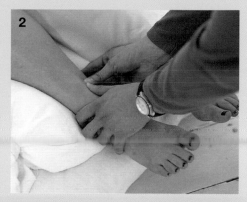

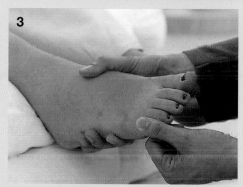

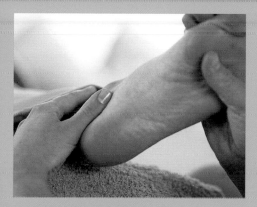

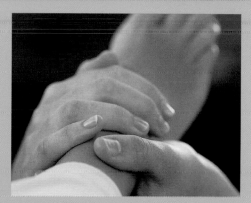

Working on the reproductive and
musculoskeletal systems

General soothing foot massage

Late pregnancy

In this stage of pregnancy, you may be troubled more by mood swings; in addition, backache due to weight gain will be further aggravated by the muscle-relaxing effects of the hormone progesterone, and insomnia is very common. The reflexology sequence featured here will help with all these conditions – practise it once a day, applying more pressure to the pituitary reflex, which produces oxytocin, the hormone that causes the womb to contract during labour and stimulates the flow of breast milk.

Quick fix

This quick and easy massage will help rejuvenate aching feet:

- Put both thumbs together on top of the foot and gradually spread them apart, applying a medium pressure, then squeeze the foot to finish. Use a soothing peppermint foot lotion for additional benefit.

Reflexology

Pre-birth sequence

1 To work on the pituitary/oxytocin reflex, support one thumb with your other hand, then use your working thumb to apply pressure to the centre of the thumb (see page 20).

2 To work on the thyroid reflex, place your hand palm downwards and support one thumb in the other hand (see page 21). Use your working thumb to walk between the two creases of the thumb. You should be stimulating the half of the thumb that is closest to the index finger.

3 To work on the uterus and ovaries reflex, turn your hand palm downwards, then use your working thumb and index finger to follow down from your thumb and little finger. Apply pressure to the small indentation at either side of the base of the wrist.

4 To work on the spine reflex use your working thumb to walk along the bone starting at the base of the thumb. Make 12 small steps along the bone to the edge of the wrist, then continue to the base of the hand.

Shiatsu

These are two particularly useful massage techniques during labour, helping to relieve the pain and bring on the contractions.

- Using the thumbs, apply strong pressure to the sacrum, the triangular bone at the base of the spine – there are four pairs of sacral points that lie in two vertical rows on either side of the spine (see page 71).

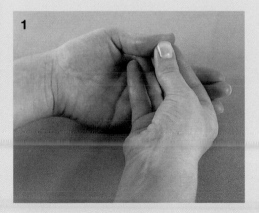

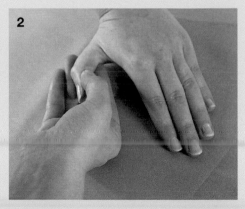

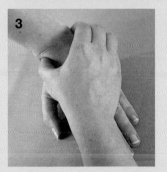

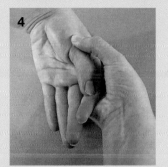

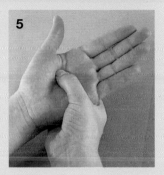

5 To work on the kidney/adrenals reflex, support one hand in the other, then place your working thumb in the webbing between the thumb and the index finger halfway down the hand. Use your thumb to hook into the webbing and apply pressure.

- Work on Bl 60, at the back of the ankle, and Sp 6, four finger-widths up the inner leg from the ankle bone, starting from the fleshy area behind the ankle bone (see page 25). Also apply pressure to tender points on the ear.

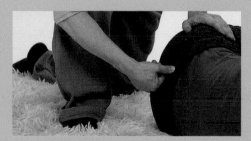

Thumbing the sacral points

Menopause

During all stages of the menopause, hormonal imbalance is to blame for symptoms that include sweating, hot flushes, migraines and bloating. There are trigger points in the abdominal wall that can bring relief – in contrast to abdominal massage, which can sometimes increase blood pressure and produce hot flushes. Gentle massage is ideal for reducing the musculoskeletal pain that is sometimes a characteristic of the menopause.

Quick fixes

Try the following simple strategies to help cope with the menopause day to day:

- Use a ribbed wooden foot roller to give your soles a speedy invigorating massage.

- Use the effleurage stroke with a luxurious oil, such as avocado, to massage the skin and at the same time nourish it and reduce dryness.

- Use the kneading technique on the thighs and hips to reduce water retention.

Western massage

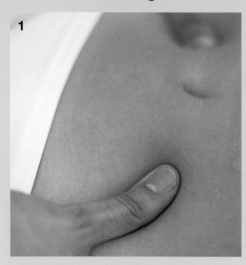

Gentle abdominal treatment

1 Place the pads of your thumbs about 7 cm (3 in) on either side of the navel and, using your body weight, lean in towards the navel and hold for five seconds. Repeat this process two or three times.

Acupressure

These acupressure points are particularly useful for combating hot flushes and other symptoms:

- Work on Sp 6, four finger-widths up the inner leg from the ankle bone, starting from the fleshy area behind the ankle bone (see page 25). Also work on Liv 3, between the big and second toes, two finger-widths up the foot from the join between the toes, and Pc 6, three finger-widths down from the wrist, pressing with the third finger, right in the centre (see page 24).

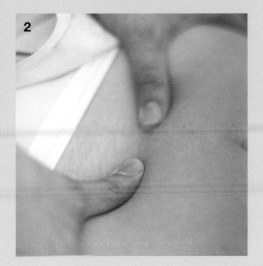

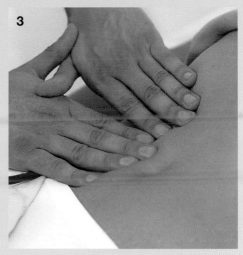

2 Move your thumbs close together and, using the pads, work as in Step 1 downwards in a straight line from just below the navel to end level with the hips, then work back up, finishing where Step 1 began. This will relax stomach tension and reduce spasms and fatigue.

3 Using very light effleurage strokes and with your hands relaxed and close together, place them on the mid-abdomen, level with the navel, and work gently in an arc towards the groin and return. Make sure that you massage both sides of the abdomen equally.

- Point Ki 1, also known as the 'bubbling spring', is in the centre of the foot, just below the ball in the middle, where the two parts meet. Work on this point while rotating the ankle.

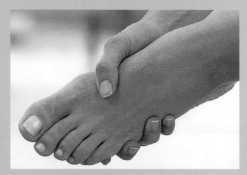

Working on the 'bubbling spring' ▶

Reflexology

Pay particular attention to the following points to help yourself or a friend through the transition.

- Work on the reproductive system, on the side of your foot in the area between the back of the heel and ankle bone, and the thyroid, on the top of the foot at the base of the big toe (see page 19).

- Work on the uterus or prostate point, which is midway between the ankle bone and the tip of the heel, on the Achilles tendon, known as the 'chronic helper', the ovaries, on the outer side of the heel, the liver, on the sole, as well as the eliminatory parts of the digestive and urinary systems to prevent constipation.

Staying positive

Desite all the negative press that the menopause receives, this can be a time of liberating, exhilarating change. Some women even find that hot flushes – or 'power surges' – clear their heads! So expect the best, not the worst, and use self-massage to help you through any bad patches that do occur.

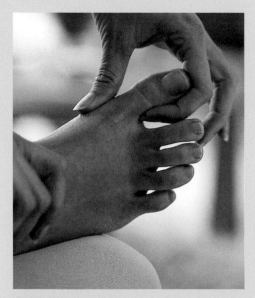

Working on the thyroid

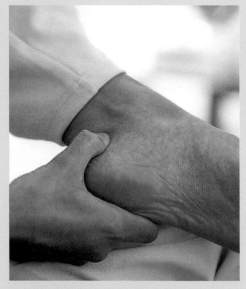

Working on the uterus

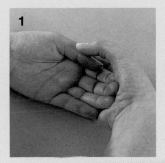

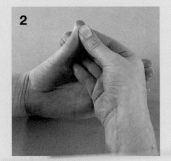

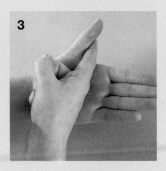

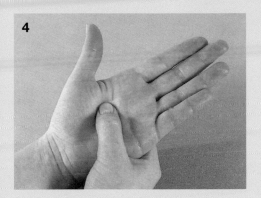

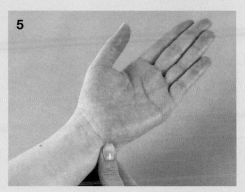

Daily menopause therapy

1 Cup one hand in the other so that your thumb rests between your index and middle fingers and use your working thumb to walk along the bone of the supported thumb from the first to the second joint. Continue to walk along the bone from the second joint to the base of the hand.

2 Support one thumb on the fingers of your other hand and use your working thumb to apply pressure and stimulate the centre of your other thumb.

3 Support your thumb as shown and place your working index finger against the first joint of the inner section of the thumb. Hook up against the bone and stimulate in clockwise or anticlockwise circles.

4 Support one hand in the other and place your working thumb in the webbing between the thumb and index finger just above the thumb muscle halfway down the hand. Use your thumb to hook into the webbing and apply pressure.

5 To work on the ovaries reflex, place your hand palm upwards and use your working index finger to follow down from the little finger to the base of the wrist where you will find a small indentation. Using the rotation-on-a-point technique, rotating alternately clockwise and anticlockwise continually, apply pressure to the point with your index finger.

Cystitis

Cystitis is a bacterial infection of the lining of the bladder, resulting in inflammation. Symptoms include painful urination, and the frequent and urgent desire to urinate. If left untreated, it can lead to a serious kidney infection.

Quick fixes

Try working on the following points to bring relief from discomfort:

- Stimulate Cv 3 on the midline of the belly, four thumb-widths below the navel.

- Apply pressure to Bl 60, on the outside of the ankle. Never stimulate this point during pregnancy.

Reflexology

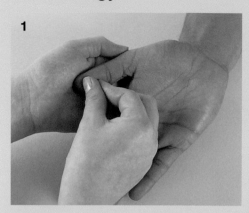

1

Massage of urinary reflexes

1 To work on the pituitary reflex, support the receiver's thumb in the palm of your hand and use your working thumb and index finger to simultaneously stimulate the centre and outside edge of the thumb (see page 20).

2 To work on the bladder reflex, support the hand across the base of the fingers and place your working thumb in the base of the muscle of the thumb, then tear down towards the wrist and stimulate.

3 To work on the ureter reflex, find the base of the receiver's lifeline, which starts at the centre of the palm just above the wrist. Use your working thumb to thumb-walk along this line and finish when you come to the webbing.

4 To work on the kidney/adrenal glands reflex, place your working thumb in the webbing between the thumb and index finger just above the thumb muscle halfway down the hand. Use your thumb to hook into the webbing and apply pressure.

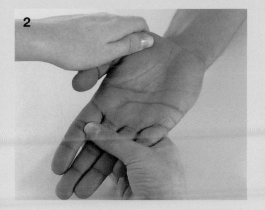

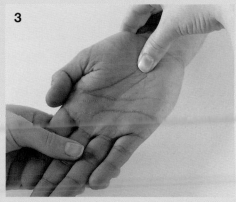

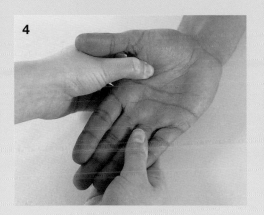

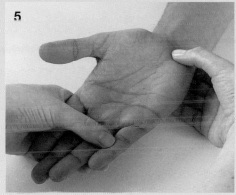

5 To work the lower back reflex, place your working thumb at the base of the receiver's hand just above the wrist and thumb-walk along the bone towards the base of the thumb. Make five small steps to the edge of the hand, stimulating with small circles at each step.

Acupressure

Target these two acupressure points to help tackle the problem of cystitis:

- Work on point St 29, which lies a hand-width below the navel, two thumb-widths out (see page 24).

- Work on point Sp 6, which is located four finger-widths up the inner leg from the ankle bone, starting from the fleshy area behind the ankle bone (but do not use this point during pregnancy).

Index

Acknowledgements

PICTURE ACKNOWLEDGEMENTS

Special Photography:
©**Octopus Publishing Group Limited**/Mike Prior.

Other photography:
Octopus Publishing Group Limited/Peter Myers 39 top right, 39 bottom right, 96 top, 96 bottom, 104 top, 104 bottom, 108; /Peter Pugh-Cook 16 top, 16 centre, 16 bottom, 21 top, 27 top, 32 left, 32 right, 33 top, 33 centre, 33 bottom, 46 top centre, 46 top left, 46 centre left, 46 centre right, 46 top right, 47 top, 47 bottom, 55 centre, 55 bottom, 56 top, 56 bottom, 57 top left, 57 top right, 57 bottom left, 60, 61, 62, 63 bottom right, 63 bottom left, 65 bottom, 67 top centre, 67 top left, 67 centre left, 67 top right, 67 centre right, 70 top right, 73 centre right, 73 bottom right, 77 bottom right, 77 bottom left, 78 left, 78 right, 79 top left, 79 top right, 79 bottom right, 83 top centre, 83 top left, 83 top right, 85 bottom right, 92 left, 92 right, 93 top left, 93 top right, 93 bottom right, 94, 95 bottom, 100 top, 100 centre, 100 bottom, 101 top, 101 bottom, 103 top centre, 103 top left, 103 centre left, 103 top right, 103 centre right, 103 bottom right, 109 top centre, 109 top left, 109 top right, 111 centre left, 111 centre, 111 centre right, 111 bottom right, 111 bottom left, 117 top left, 117 centre left, 117 top right, 117 centre, 117 centre right, 121 top centre, 121 top left, 121 centre left, 121 top right, 121 centre right, 122, 123 top left, 123 top right, 123 bottom right, 123 bottom left; /Gareth Sambidge 4 top right, 5, 7, 8, 12, 13 top, 13 centre, 13 bottom, 45 top left, 45 top right, 45 top centre right, 45 top centre left, 59 top left, 59 top right, 59 bottom right, 59 bottom left, 68, 69 top left, 69 centre left, 69 top right, 69 centre right, 74 top centre, 74 top left, 74 top right, 74 bottom right, 77 top centre, 77 top left, 77 top right, 81 top left, 81 centre left, 81 top right, 81 centre right, 81 bottom right, 81 bottom left, 84, 85 top left, 85 top right, 88 top, 88 bottom, 89 top, 89 bottom, 91 top centre, 91 top left, 91 top right, 95 top left, 95 top right, 97 top left, 99 top left, 99 top right, 107 bottom right, 115 top left, 115 top right, 115 centre right, 118, 119 top left, 119 top right; /Ian Wallace 1, 2, 4 bottom right, 15 top left, 15 top right, 15 bottom right, 15 bottom left, 18, 19 top, 19 bottom, 20 top, 20 bottom, 21 bottom, 22 left, 22 right, 24, 25 left, 25 right, 40 top, 40 centre, 41 top, 43 top centre, 43 top left, 43 centre, 43 top right, 43 centre right, 43 bottom right, 43 bottom left, 45 bottom right, 45 bottom left, 49 right, 49 top left, 49 bottom left, 50 top, 50 bottom, 51 top, 51 bottom, 52, 53 top left, 53 top right, 53 bottom right, 53 bottom left, 54, 55 top, 64, 65 top, 70 centre left, 70 bottom left, 73 top centre, 73 top left, 73 top right, 82 centre left, 82 bottom left, 83 bottom right, 86, 87 top, 87 bottom, 98, 99 bottom right, 99 bottom left, 105 left, 105 top right, 105 centre right, 106, 107 top left, 107 centre left, 109 bottom right, 110 top left, 110 top right, 110 bottom right, 112 left, 112 right, 115 bottom right, 115 bottom left, 119 bottom right, 120 left, 120 right; /Jacqui Wornell 3, 26 left, 26 right, 27 bottom, 28 left, 28 right, 29 left, 29 right, 38 top, 38 bottom, 39 top left, 39 bottom left, 63 top left, 63 top right.

Executive Editor **Jane McIntosh**
Editor **Charlotte Wilson**
Executive Art Editor **Darren Southern**
Designer **Lisa Tai**
Production Controller **Nigel Reed**
Picture Researcher **Jennifer Veall**